D0587138

A WHITE EAGLE LODGE
BOOK OF HEALTH AND HEALING

By the same author

—

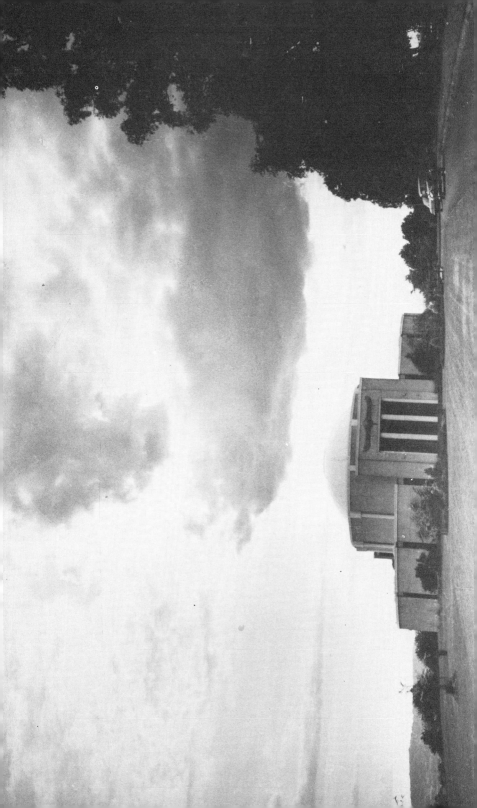

A WHITE EAGLE LODGE

BOOK OF HEALTH AND HEALING

JOAN HODGSON

THE WHITE EAGLE PUBLISHING TRUST
NEW LANDS : LISS : HAMPSHIRE : ENGLAND

First published 1983
First paperback edition 1985
Reprinted 1993

© Joan Hodgson, 1983

British Library Cataloguing in Publication Data

Hodgson, Joan

A White Eagle Lodge book of health and healing
1. Spiritual healing and spiritualism
I. Title
615.8'52   BF1275.F3
ISBN 0-85487-070-9

The quotation from MAN'S SUPREME INHERITANCE *is reprinted by kind
permission of Associated Book Publishers Ltd; that from* Here's Health *by
kind permission of Newman Turner Publications Ltd; and that from* YOUR
DAILY BREAD *by kind permission of Faber & Faber Ltd.*

.

Set in 11 on 13pt Baskerville
by Waveney Typesetters, Norwich
and printed in Great Britain
by Cambridge University Press

CONTENTS

LIST OF ILLUSTRATIONS

*The frontispiece is by Robert Reding and no. 8 by Colum
Hayward. All other photographs by Bruce Clarke.*

PREFACE

THE WHITE EAGLE LODGE was founded by Grace and Ivan Cooke in 1936, in premises in Pembroke Gardens, London W8. The instructions given by White Eagle at that time were clear and precise. His workers were to find a centre in London from which the teachings could be given forth. His workers must go forward in faith, doing everything in their power to create a church, beautiful, peaceful and harmonious, which would always maintain an atmosphere of kindliness. So only could the teachings of the Wise Ones in spirit be given to humanity in preparation for the time of its greatest need. It was recognised that this venture would require some courage, but the assurance was given that so long as his workers were loyal and faithful to their calling, all that was necessary would be provided.

The basis upon which this church was to be built was that of the family – of the family spirit wide enough to embrace all comers. White Eagle said that only in a united family could there be found sufficient harmony, love and understanding, upon which to base this church, which was to become like a lighthouse in a storm-tossed world – a world in which a dire battle would be waged between the forces of the light and the principalities and powers of darkness.

The family were to create a home in London, a spiritual home to which all could come who were unhappy, bereaved, lonely or puzzled by life and its seeming injustices. In an atmosphere of love, understanding and spiritual benediction, souls were to be healed, comforted and given light. Nothing was to stand in the way of the gradual building of this spiritual centre of power and light, which would help those on earth to glimpse the harmony of the heavenly world.

From small beginnings, the work of White Eagle, through Grace Cooke his medium, grew and flourished. Healing prayer groups were started and healers trained in the 'laying on of hands'. White Eagle and his medium worked unceasingly, giving a continual stream of inspired teachings, most of which are now available in book form through the White Eagle Publishing Trust. He trained his students in spiritual unfoldment, and he led them in the healing work, diagnosing the cause of patients' 'dis-ease' and specifying the colours that were to be directed to the psychic centres or chakras in treatment. Ivan Cooke protected and supported his wife in her work, which required great sensitivity of her, and became the first great exponent of the White Eagle healing (see his book *Healing by the Spirit*, White Eagle Publishing Trust, 1976).

Pembroke Hall was bombed early in the 'Blitz' and in faith White Eagle's family were led to other premises in the same district, larger and more accessible, and yet quiet and at an unusually low rental. The manifest advantages of the move have always been an example to followers of the work of how good comes out of evil, and of the guidance of spirit. The new premises, 9 and 9a St Mary Abbots Place, London W8, remain the London quarters of the work today. The Lodge was restarted by sheer hard work; and after the War, by the combined efforts of Mr and Mrs Cooke and their immediate family and the generosity of White Eagle's larger family, these Kensington premises were purchased over a long period, and also a country centre, 'a fair place with a fair name' as White Eagle predicted, New Lands, near Liss in Hampshire.

It is necessary to devote a few words to Mr and Mrs Cooke's family. Joan, the elder daughter, gave up her work as a teacher during the war to devote herself to the inner teaching and healing work of the Lodge. She married John Hodgson in 1943 and he later took on the responsibilities of Treasurer of the Lodge. Ylana Hayward, her sister, was by White Eagle given the task from the commencement of the work of being its organising secretary.

Before all the mortgages and loans on the Lodge properties were fully cleared, White Eagle laid before his medium and the family a vision of the White Temple on New Lands hill, from which rays of Light, healing and peace would radiate across the world. In 1974 this Temple became a physical reality, again built by the faith and generosity of members and friends, the wider family of the Lodge. Its purpose is truly to create a sanctuary, a meeting place between earth and spirit.

This was the culmination of Grace and Ivan Cooke's life's work, after which they gradually withdrew, leaving Joan and Ylana to continue, with the love and co-operation of their families, a new generation of whom were by then supporting the work. Jenny Dent has since become General Secretary and her husband Geoffrey is Treasurer (John Hodgson taking over from Joan as Healing Secretary); while Rose Elliot, Joan's other daughter, helped to bring about a small revolution in eating habits in Britain with her vegetarian cookery books, of which *Simply Delicious* (1967) and three others were published by the White Eagle Publishing Trust. The efforts of Ylana's husband Geoffrey had been vital in setting professional standards in editing and production in the White Eagle publications; and it is in this area, the publications, that their sons Colum and Jeremy are now most concerned.

On 3 September 1979 Grace Cooke left the physical life, shortly after midnight, and before many hours had passed made her radiant, loving presence clearly seen and felt by her two daughters and other members of her family. There

3

could be no sorrow, because there truly was no separation. Trained and disciplined over the years in building a 'bridge of light' between the two worlds we were all aware that the loving wise Mother of the whole work was much more active than when she had been hampered by a weary physical body. She soon demonstrated in many ways that she was still caring not only for her personal family, but her wider family all over the world.

After his wife's passing, it seemed as if quite a large part of Ivan's soul went with her, for he seemed largely unaware that her physical presence had gone. He settled down to a peaceful existence, sleeping much of the time; but when he was awake, he radiated such gentleness and sweetness of spirit that all who were close to him felt the blessing of his presence and tended his physical needs with loving devotion. He passed into the light on the evening of 28 July 1981, just as the first beacon was lighted in celebration of the wedding of the Prince and Princess of Wales.

The Golden Jubilee of the White Eagle Lodge is now approaching. For nearly fifty years his students have been doing their best to put into practice White Eagle's teachings about healthy and harmonious living and the joy of true communion between the two worlds. He once told us that the real proof of spirit was not in isolated manifestations of psychic power, which could only be repeated under certain conditions. The life of the spirit, the wonderful guidance of the spirit, must be demonstrated in every aspect of the life.

Over the years we have watched this working out in our own lives and the lives of many who have been blessed and healed by the power of the spirit and inspired by the White Eagle teachings, which give courage and strength to meet the challenges and trials of mortal existence, and by the wonderful hope and joy which grows in the heart as we learn the truth of communion of spirit.

This book is dedicated with love and heartfelt gratitude to

our beloved three in the world of spirit: White Eagle, Grace and Ivan Cooke.

The White Eagle Lodge Prayer of Dedication

May the light of Christ shining in my heart stand guard over my thoughts and guide my speech and actions into ways of service.

May the light of Christ shine from my heart
    To heal the sick in mind and body;
    To comfort the bereaved;
    To sustain the weary.

May the light of Christ illumine my understanding and the understanding of all men, bringing true vision and awareness of the eternal life, and of the Christ within all mankind.

The reader of this book is also directed to White Eagle's own words on healing, given in the book *Heal Thyself* (White Eagle Publishing Trust, 1962).

1

THE LIFE THAT MAKES ALL
THINGS NEW

EVEN BEFORE the White Eagle Lodge came into being White Eagle started training a small group in spiritual unfoldment, training them to realise that deep within their hearts, beneath all the turmoil of the everyday consciousness, was a different self, a self based in eternity, which was always peaceful, steady and still. This deep eternal self, like a light shining in the darkness of the physical life, could with training and discipline of the outer self become so powerful and bright that it could awaken new life in the cells of the human body. That light of the eternal self could be likened to the Pole Star as it guides the traveller through the darkness and illumines for each man his own path of life. Week by week, White Eagle trained his group of devotees in the art of stilling the outer mind and becoming aware of this light of the spirit, which could be strengthened and directed as a healing force: a power for good which could help not only sick and sad individuals but whole nations and their leaders. Constantly White Eagle stressed the need to discipline mind and body so that both would become more responsive, clearer channels through which this inner light, the saving grace of the Christ, could shine.

The name White Eagle symbolises a spiritual teacher. In the Christian tradition the White Eagle is the symbol of St John, the disciple of Love who was so close to the Master Jesus, and whose influence is becoming increasingly prominent as humanity goes forward into the Aquarian Age. The first chapter of his gospel deals with the Light, the Word of God in man which dwells in the darkness of matter and which eventually is destined to permeate and glorify all physical life, raising it from darkness to light.

White Eagle told his students that during the latter part of this century there would be a great surge forward both in scientific and spiritual knowledge so that humanity would be ready to accept spiritual truths which at that time it just could not understand. This is now happening, for there is no doubt that the climate of spiritual understanding is now very different from what it was in the 1930s; especially among young people, so many of whom are ready to accept the fact of the inner life of the spirit. The study of alternative medicine, the paranormal, extra-sensory perception, occultism, astrology and magic, fascinates many, and in the United States such subjects are already researched in the university thesis.

On the outer planes the 1930s were the years of the steady build-up towards the Second World War, but on the inner planes preparations had long been made to help humanity through the conflict ahead, which involved not only battles on the physical plane but a tremendous confrontation of the forces of good and evil – of principalities and powers of darkness with the angels of Light. This was the period of the great guides of Spiritualism, especially the four teachers Red Cloud, White Hawk, Silver Birch and White Eagle. The four worked closely in harmony, although the mission of each was different. Together they worked, each at his own level, to awaken mankind from its limited materialistic outlook. There was a tremendous effort from the world of spirit to break through the hard crust of thinking which pandered only to the demands of the body and the lower mind.

Although the mediums of these four beloved teachers are now themselves in the world of light, we know that they still continue their work as part of the Shining Army in the invisible world who are dedicated to the task of bringing humanity through the difficult transition which always occurs between the different astrological ages, the Months of the Great Year. For we are now nearing the end of the Piscean Age and responding with rapidly increasing momentum to the mental stimulation of the new Age of Aquarius. Inevitably the old religions which have upheld humanity during the past few centuries seem outdated and outworn. The old forms of worship to many people seem stereotypes, almost as if the light has been withdrawn from the creeds and dogmas which have formed a scaffolding for the soul-temple of humanity during the Piscean Age. These periods of transition between the astrological ages always appear to bring chaos, when on the outer plane all the old order seems to be turned upside down. The discoveries of scientists and the way their findings have been interpreted in the press have caused many people to discard their religious beliefs. This means that in all the problems of their personal lives, and in their anxieties about the world, they have no spiritual support to turn to. Without faith in a divine order, without knowledge of the wonderful law which governs life, which manifests throughout nature and is so clearly demonstrated in the cosmic order of the stars and planets, without such understanding, life can indeed be frightening and bleak.

While people still have a faith in God, they have the comfort of prayer, even if this prayer is only a childlike petition to a Being in the sky. The ability to reach out in prayer – a true sincere turning of the thoughts to a Being who is all-loving, all-powerful and all-understanding of human need – is an inestimable blessing; for as soon as the soul makes an effort to reach out to this infinite Power, the inner light is stimulated and healing begins. This simple faith has sustained great men, leaders, teachers, artists, scientists and healers throughout the centuries.

The essence of White Eagle's work throughout the years has been to awaken mankind to the light of the spirit. It is the purpose of all the books, the lectures, the services, the training groups and healing work of the White Eagle Lodge.

Within every one of us, he says, there are two centres of consciousness: the mind in the head, which is needed for our work in the outer world and for the practical care and maintenance of the body; and the mind in the heart, that peaceful inner light through which we can hold communion with the eternal world, and which is needed for the care and development of the soul. It is neglect of this contact with the inner light that allows it so quickly to be overlaid and smothered with the cares, the problems, the excitements and the pleasures of the outer world. Within every human being there is a constant struggle between the self of the earth and the true inner flame which is the guide of every soul through eternity.

Strangely enough, one of the causes of the stress problems of the present day seems to be the very diversity of opportunities for gaining mental knowledge. This tremendous stimulation of the outer mind, together with speed of communication, is one of the blessings and one of the curses of the New Age. We cannot hold back the flow of knowledge and the quickening tempo of life any more than we can hold back the incoming tide; but we all need to find a way of adjusting to the quickening pace and using rather than being used by the variety of new technology which is transforming our everyday lives. Although in many ways physical life has been made easier by modern inventions, they have also made it more difficult (because of their hold on the head-mind) to hold fast to the inner light of the spirit. This light can so quickly be buried by the cares and interests of daily life that until some crisis comes we give no thought to the source of our life, health and well-being. Even minimal contact with the divine light, such as a brief grace before meals, at one time brought people momentarily into contact with the deeper self, so that somehow we knew that the framework of faith was there to be called upon in times of deep need.

For those who are awakened to the truth of the inner light there is the problem of the multiplicity of spiritual paths and spiritual teachers. The student who prides himself on being open-minded and ready to study anything eventually finds himself either cynical about everything, or else in a complete muddle because of the differing opinions of the various groups and teachers. White Eagle prophesied that this would be the case, as the new ideas and desire for psychic development symptomatic of the Aquarian Age began to be more widespread. He always insisted that those who wanted to unfold their spiritual awareness should find a teacher with whom they felt in harmony and follow with loyalty and devotion the path of that one teacher.

In the study of spiritual truth there is a wide difference between the stimulation of the mind, which comes through studying books, however spiritual their content, and the stimulation of the true inner light, which comes in the deep stillness of prayer and meditation. The practice of meditation is becoming more widespread; but here again some discrimination is needed, for in meditation we seek entrance to an inner world which is much more real than the average person realises, and people who start to follow this path in lighthearted ignorance or seeking sensation can soon find themselves having experiences they cannot control.

Just as the physical body has a natural inclination for certain comforts and sensations, the soul-body also reaches out with desire and greed for knowledge and sensation; and can become just as clogged with too much food as can the physical body. There is a sloth and gluttony of the soul quite as surely as of the body. Of all the temptations of the present age, perhaps this is one of those most responsible for ill-health and nervous strain in our civilisation.

Little children, when they start to paint, are given a few

11

basic colours. They splodge them on to the paper with abandon and quite soon have a murky mess of paint which has run together in a peculiar grey-black effect. As the children grow older and learn how to use the colours in a certain order, and to wait until they are dry before applying another, they begin to produce beautiful pictures. The same principle applies to those who want to tread a path of spiritual unfoldment. If they try to follow every teacher, they will finish like the young children: with a murky splodge of mental and spiritual confusion instead of a clear, bright picture.

The White Eagle Lodge is a mystery school offering a path of spiritual unfoldment which is simple and safe. It is based entirely on devotion to the inner light, to disciplining the outer life so that this light is strengthened and becomes a source of joy, courage and inspiration through the humdrum problems of everyday living. More than this, it can bring healing, comfort and peace to our family, friends and co-workers.

White Eagle has given certain principles of healthy living which he assured us could transform our daily lives. The light of the spirit, the shining higher self, can only function on the physical plane through the mechanism of the body, the brain and the five senses. The body is the instrument, the temple of the spirit. Any musician knows the importance of a beautiful instrument if he is to express fully the message of the music. Every artist is dependent on the quality of his materials. In the same way the quality of our response to the power of the spirit is dependent on how the body feels.

In childhood and youth many people enjoy an abundance of health, a vitality and energy which they take for granted. It is only as the misuse of energy and over-indulgence of bodily appetites causes health troubles that they begin to realise that certain discipline is required if they are to maintain a healthy body into maturity and old age. Good health, in adulthood, does not just happen. It is partly a question of environment and the type of life that circumstances force us to lead, but also it is a question of knowledge; of the ability to adjust to circumstances and of exercising the self-discipline required to put into practice certain very simple principles which if faithfully followed will help us to make our bodies better instruments for service and for the full enjoyment of all the beauty that life on the physical plane has to offer.

This inner light, the life that makes all things new, will only grow bright and shining as we give time and attention to it. To be healthy and strong in the light means that we are learning to drink from the eternal spring, the living water which can heal and renew the cells of the body. Then, as true children of the new Age of Aquarius, we try to give the water of life, the comfort of true spiritual communion, to our companions.

2

THE BODY OF LIGHT, THE
SOLAR BODY AND THE
BODY-ELEMENTAL

A T SOME TIME WE ALL have to learn that we are not the physical body although we have to function through it. We have a number of subtler bodies, which infiltrate the physical cells as water infiltrates a sponge. We have a mind body which colours all our thinking, and a feeling body through which emotions are expressed. While these subtler bodies are only visible to a clairvoyant, their quality can be felt in the aura which radiates from the physical body. Even more subtle than the mental and emotional bodies is that which some people term the higher mind, which is of still finer texture than the others and is like a ladder up which we can ascend in consciousness right into the heavenly spheres.

All these subtler vehicles are able to manifest through the physical by means of the etheric body, which is like a bridge between the visible and the invisible world. All natural form, physical form, has an etheric counterpart; and the inner worlds to which the soul withdraws at death are composed of varying grades of this etheric matter. Etheric matter varies in its degree of subtlety according to its plane of manifestation, but it is the substance of creation, from the first breathing forth from the Sun, the Source, the Flame, which is clad in many layers, from the finest to the coarsest, namely dense physical matter. We all have an etheric body which is a finer replica of the physical body, and is also closely attuned to all the subtler bodies. Attuned to the physical body, the etheric can even be glimpsed by some people, as a pale indigo shadow standing out about an inch

14

from the physical. It is closely allied with the grey matter of the brain and the nervous system. In the etheric body are vibrant energy centres linked to the physical body through the ductless glands and also through the chief nerve ganglia.

Each of the subtler bodies has its special link with the physical at one of these energy centres, known in eastern philosophy as the chakras. During the course of evolution all the chakras will be brought into full manifestation, as the deep eternal self of every individual learns how to control and use them. Just as a baby has to learn stage by stage how to use its faculties of movement and speech and has to learn how to interpret the various impressions which come through the five senses, so man's real eternal self gradually learns to bring into full manifestation the spiritual faculties, which will in time illumine each of the bodies in which it is clothed. In every incarnation we come back into a physical body with a certain task, certain opportunities for developing a facet of our spiritual consciousness. White Eagle teaches that the particular facet which is to be developed during the present incarnation is shown astrologically by the position of the sun in the horoscope (shown by the date of birth). The sun traditionally signifies the heart-centre or chakra, the one which links us with that inmost place where dwells the true self.

Incarnation by incarnation we are all building the temple of our soul, that body of light which White Eagle often refers to as the solar body. He tells us (in an unpublished teaching), 'Every living soul on earth is in a physical body in order to build and create, in due time, that body of light which the ancient brotherhoods called the solar body. When you are blessed with the gift of clear vision or clairvoyance, you will be able to see that solar body in your brother man just above his physical form. Within or above every man, woman (yes, and child too), if they have reached a certain level of spiritual development or evolution, is to be seen this

15

beautiful solar body, or body of light created out of the light of the Son, the Christos. We are not speaking of an orthodox individual person. We are speaking of the Son of the Father–Mother God, the pure white light which is in the Son and which descends to the earth from its Creator. Bear our words in mind and think about them, because there is a deeper truth here than the words at first convey. The Son of God is the heavenly light of the Sun and is the Creator; and every living thing is permeated with the Son and with the Light.'

This pure white flame of the living Christ – the Sun-God in every man – to grow and gain experience seeks to manifest in form. To do this it must, through the will, or energy, which is divine thought, draw together and shape the surrounding ether. Just as in a seed the root first goes down to the earth to draw in nourishment, and then takes form through the shaping of the leaves, the flower, and the fruit of the plant, so the divine will creates from the experiences in earth, in the heaviest, darkest form of etheric substance, the vehicles it needs to function on the different planes of being: develops the roots, the leaves, the flowers, the fruit. During every incarnation the experiences of each season of growth add to the beauty of what eventually becomes a glorious Tree of Life in the infinite and eternal Garden of Eden.

The pure white flame, the seed of God, the Christ within man, is in esoteric astrology symbolised by the Pole Star, the star which guides the soul throughout the long journey during which it gains control over every plane of matter. In the horoscope, until a certain stage of spiritual maturity is reached, this Pole Star of every man's being can only manifest through the Sun-sign, which indicates the particular aspect of the solar body which is being worked on during the present incarnation. So the Sun-sign at birth gives an indication of the deeper spiritual lessons of the

16

elements which the experiences of life are to teach the soul. It is this body of light, the solar body, that we gradually build through our prayer, aspiration and effort towards good thought and as we struggle with our life's problems. The solar body will then illumine the mind and emotions of the personal self, symbolised in the horoscope by the Moon; which in turn reflects the light of the Sun or solar body onto the earth, the physical body. The secret of health and healing is this illumination of the ordinary material self by the light of the innermost Sun. In Christianity this is known as the saving power of Christ. In the eastern philosophies it is *yoga* – the union of the finite and infinite. This true immortal self, the Pole Star of our being, shining in the solar body, will eventually govern and control every cell of the physical body and all the finer vehicles which interpenetrate it. The Sun is the king, the centre of the universe of the self, just as it is the centre of the solar system and stands for the central Sun of our galaxy, the Almighty, Invisible, Universal I AM . . . the spiritual Sun of all life.

White Eagle continues, 'You have been told that the great initiate, the Master Jesus, through many incarnations spent not only on earth but also in another more highly evolved planet, prepared and developed this perfect solar body or body of light through which Christ, the Son, was able to manifest. When the body of light has been created in man, the whole physical body becomes illumined, and thus a purer vehicle for the use of the soul. We are endeavouring to help you in your meditations and by the power of God-thought to develop this higher body, this body of light, the body of the Sun. This is the purpose of meditation, which is the only way in which man can consciously develop that pure body of light. This is why meditation was practised in the mystery schools and the brotherhood of all time, and why the brethren withdrew from the material life into communities or brotherhoods, dwelling in high places, raised above worldliness.' The trouble is that when the glorious eternal light shines in the darkness, the darkness literally comprehends it not. In other words, we find it difficult to disentangle our true selves from the sensations of the body, the mind and the feelings; and until we are trained to do so we think that these *are* ourselves.

All of us are to a large extent dominated by the habits of thought and feeling which we absorb unconsciously in infancy. These form the foundation upon which the rest of our lives are built. When the tiny baby is conceived in the womb it emerges from the etheric world, created from the etheric substance which has been drawn down into physical manifestation through the physical union of the father and mother. Ideally the physical union is the culmination of deep mutual love and friendship which brings a union not only of physical bodies but of all the subtler soul vehicles. Union such as this forms an etheric cradle of harmony, in which the incarnating soul can gradually come to terms with the physical environment. With every breath the newborn child absorbs the soul-life of the parents and the home environment; and for the first seven years this unconscious absorption continues. (In some cases, of course, it will be the soul-life of the person most involved with caring for the child, but we would be wrong to under-estimate the primary bond between child and parent, which is deeply karmic.)

The habits of body, mind and feelings taken on in infancy are of course later adjusted and moulded by our life-experience; but these deeply ingrained habits give us an almost automatic response to the events of daily life. We probably only realise how instinctive are our physical habits when, for instance, some minor accident to the hands forces us to change our way of cleaning teeth or combing hair. We feel completely 'cack-handed'. According to whether we are natural optimists or pessimists our mental reaction to events

18

is also fairly habitual and only shaken out of routine by some surprise or shock.

Ivan Cooke says in *Healing by the Spirit*, 'The subconscious mind should be thought of as an integral part of every human being, having been born with the babe. Perhaps it began to build the body of that babe from the moment of conception, who can say? But let us assume that with the birth of the baby, it immediately takes charge of its welfare. It directs and manipulates the internal arrangements of the child – its systems of ingestion, digestion and elimination, its breathing, its blood circulation, its very heart beat. It can prove itself very imperious, as every parent knows, when the baby feels hungry or uncomfortable. What it wants it will get, for it is a one-track mind, self-seeking and wholly egotistical in nature. It is this mind which renders the baby during its early years so self-centred a creature. Only later, when the conscious mind takes over to some extent, does a child begin to think of others and to show a degree of un-selfishness.'

White Eagle has always made a distinction between the subconscious and the superconscious mind. Both are beyond the scope of our everyday consciousness, and gradually the conscious mind will learn how to draw upon the immortal wisdom and strength of the one to control and illumine the other. He tells us in *Spiritual Unfoldment I*, 'Attached to the physical body is a certain form recognisable as the body-elemental. This is not an evil thing; it has its place in the evolution, not only of man but also of the lower forms of life. We have been asked how it is that when man is in a physical body the pull of evil seems so much stronger than the attraction, the aspiration to good. You will find the answer in this body- or desire-elemental, which is very strong in most men [and women]. Man has to learn in the course of his evolution that the higher self (which is only partially in evidence in most of us) must gain complete domination over the body-elemental. The home of the human ego is in the celestial body, the highest and purest aura of man. The bidding of the ego descends to man's consciousness as his intuition: you call it conscience. But the body-elemental is also assisting man in his evolution, as a kind of ballast which keeps him tied to earth. You all feel this pull, but it is not to be regarded as evil, for it forces growth of the spiritual or God-consciousness which we all come back on earth to unfold.'

The task before each one of us during our earth life is to learn how to bring the divine mind, the mind in the heart, into operation; how to strengthen it through regular periods of quiet contemplation so that we establish full communication between the ordinary self of every day, governed mostly by the body-mind, and the eternal shining self, the Star within, the architect of our lives. Few people in the West can manage in their busy lives of action to devote long hours to the type of meditation practised in the East. Those born into western bodies are learning through practical action, and have to find ways of making quick, habitual contact with the inner flame and expressing in more perfect action the guidance which will come from it.

The best times for strengthening the contact between the higher self – the mind in the heart – and the outer self are the periods on first waking and before settling to sleep. These are times when there is some interpenetration of the two worlds, the inner and the outer. Even five minutes of conscious attunement to the Christ Star before rising in the morning and before going to sleep at night will strengthen and hold the line of communication with the world of light. This is achieved not so much by an effort of the mind as by a conscious letting-go, by surrendering all the concerns of the outer life and opening the heart to the inflow of light, as the flower opens to the sun.

Few people realise how much a quiet firm direction of

their thoughts before settling to sleep can help them to draw strength and wisdom to control the outer mind and the body-elemental through contact with that true, eternal self, which can be symbolised as a clear, bright six-pointed star at the heart of the blazing Sun.

Before settling down for the night first make sure that the physical tensions of the body are released by the methodical stretching and relaxing of all the joints and muscles from the toes up to the head. A sequence for this is given in chapter seven. Follow the sequence until the breathing is utterly peaceful, quiet, steady and even. As you observe and listen it will become slower.

The sound of this slow even breathing is rather like the inflowing and the outflowing of the waves on the seashore, and you can easily become one with the rhythm. Feel that you are part of the eternal ocean of life, part of the waves breaking on the seashore. With every inbreath feel yourself drawing back with the waves, back and back into the heart of life, into the Sun–Star which is shining down across the sea. Become united with the glorious heart of the Sun. Then, as the outbreathing starts, the light shines from your heart, illumining the waters of the soul. You are the sun-light. The waves break on the shore, carrying the light to every grain of sand – to every cell of the body. Continue to feel this indrawing and outrushing of this great sea of life, going into the heart of the Sun–Star and flowing out re-charged with life-force. With every inbreathing the heart-centre is becoming more radiant, more sun-like. With every outbreathing the light pours forth, healing, strengthening, renewing every cell of the body. It begins to radiate far beyond the little physical body; a great Sun shining out into the world to bring healing and peace to all humanity.

You are now in a state of peaceful attunement with the higher self where the body-elemental will be beautifully receptive to commands and instructions from the higher self

– the eternal you. If you are conscious of any weakness in the body, any organ or function that needs healing, now is the time to direct the body to set the healing forces in motion. Formulate a clear direction in the outer mind, which is now attuned to the Christ self, and strengthen this by actually speaking or whispering the direction. First affirm oneness with the divine self, the I AM, by naming the special attribute which is to be suggested to the body-elemental. For instance, if there is much pain, quietly repeat the words 'I AM divine peace, divine peace, divine peace; I AM releasing all pain and tension in (name the particular part of the body); I AM divine peace, I AM releasing all pain and tension'. When there is great pain, this effort of divine will and aspiration may at first seem impossible; but peaceful, quiet perseverance with the gentle deep breathing and affirmation *will* help. It takes practice and an effort from the deepest spirit, but it is possible gradually to train the body-elemental to let go of all pain, to rise right out of it.

If strength and vitality is needed, or healing and renewal of a certain organ, concentrate on the realisation that 'The strength of glorious Sun-spirit shines through my being, healing and restoring (name the dis-eased organ)'. Repeat 'The strength', etc., then 'I AM the resurrection and the life'.

These affirmations faithfully practised can work miracles. This has been proved on many occasions by those with patience and persistence to 'keep on keeping on', as White Eagle puts it. If the body is slow to respond to the direction do not give up but try to formulate the directions a little more clearly at the moment when the body and mind feel completely relaxed, just before settling to sleep. The more sleepy and relaxed the outer mind, the more clearly can the higher mind give the direction to the subconscious self, while with the gentle breathing you keep your whole being open to the Sun–Star.

Strong, clear affirmations can be used to help the body-elemental overcome addiction to smoking, drugs or alcohol provided that deep down the soul really wants to be free of these addictions. In such cases, having established the contact with the eternal self through the relaxation and quiet breathing, quietly formulate the thought 'Every cell of my being is filled with light . . . filled with light . . . releasing me from all desire for (tobacco, alcohol, etc.), I am letting it go . . . letting it go . . . letting it go'. Repeat the mantram. It is important that you formulate the direction clearly and exactly, strengthening the attunement with the shining, eternal self as you do so. Make each affirmation clearly and firmly, but in a peaceful, relaxed way three times, then let it be. Continue the peaceful 'seashore breathing' until you feel the inclination to turn into your usual sleep-position.

Try to adjust your waking time so that you can allow a little time for the soul to re-establish contact with the physical world. If you wake so late that you are forced to leap out of bed and scurry through your preparations for the day, you quickly cut yourself off from your lifeline, your line of light with the eternal self. Give yourself time to lie on your back stretching and relaxing joints and muscles, as at night, until you give one or two good yawns which thoroughly relax your shoulders and ribs and enable you to breathe more freely. Before getting out of bed, just give yourself a minute or two for quiet breathing, again feeling that with each breath you are absorbing into your heart the glorous light of the eternal Sun, source of all health, strength and wisdom.

> 'Breathe on me, Breath of God,
>   Fill me with life anew,
> That I may love what thou dost love,
>   And do what thou wouldst do.'

Hold in your thoughts the glory of the Sun and its life-giving healing power, and from your heart pray for strength and wisdom for the day ahead. Then quietly proceed with your morning's work.

Although these two routines sound simple and easy, it takes will-power and perseverance to develop them into a habit as automatic as cleaning the teeth and other physical routines. But even the busiest person should be able to adjust their lives to take in these few minutes of quiet at each end of the day. In the days of strict religious observance, many children were trained to kneel and say their prayers night and morning. These routines are a more comfortable method of attuning the outer self to the inner light, and if practised with understanding and real aspiration will prove over months and years of practice to be extraordinarily helpful. They are helping to strengthen and build the solar body and to bring the light of the innermost spirit into outer manifestation.

White Eagle asks his students to attune themselves to the Christ Star and to radiate the light to all humanity at the magical hours of 3, 6, 9 and 12, the hours which on a circular clock form the points of a cross within the circle, a magical symbol of ancient origin. This for many people is a great effort, but again it is well worth persevering because each time we try to make the contact with that inner light, that eternal Pole Star of our being, we are strengthening the conscious link with the body of light. Eventually it will help us to function in full consciousness on any plane of being; and enable us in time, after many lives, to raise the very physical atoms. White Eagle says (in another teaching), 'There comes a time when the solar force so interpenetrates the physical body that its deadness and earthiness gradually falls away, gradually dies – dust to dust, ashes to ashes. These words are in your burial service. We want to give a more beautiful outlook. We want you to understand that this refers not just to the disintegration of a physical body that you know and love. It has a far deeper meaning. This is the gradual falling-away of those atoms which are of the earth, earthy; but there are spiritual atoms which at the same time are entering the physical body and gradually re-creating it and making it a body of light, a true solar body. Instead of being subject to disease and decay it has entered into eternal life. *I give unto them eternal life.* This is the real meaning of what Jesus Christ said, and is the truth of all time. Man's body will be revivified, re-created, glorified by the Solar Logos. Thus there will be no more death, no more ''wailing and gnashing of teeth'', no more sorrow because man will have entered into the full glory of his being, that which was intended for him when the world began; man will have entered into the Promised Land.'

MORE ABOUT STAR-BREATHING

REGULAR PRACTICE of what we will hence-forth call Star-breathing is the greatest possible help in strengthening conscious contact with the heart-mind, the mind of the true self through which we can bring harmony into our individual lives. Most people long to attain poise; long for a tranquillity of mind and heart which remains unruffled by the frets and strains of daily life. To contact one who is so poised is always a joy, for under such an influence we find our own restless minds growing peaceful. In a state of peace we accomplish more with less expenditure of nervous energy and effort. Such souls are rare, for the general rush of modern life will wear down even the strongest nervous system unless we can discover the secret of constant renewal. So many people drive themselves to keep going until sickness or a breakdown enforces that complete rest which nature needs to replace the squandered reserves of strength and energy.

It is easy to waste a great deal of energy without accom-plishing much when we fail to control and organise our faculties. We mean to do certain jobs – to write a letter, phone a friend, fix something which is broken – but before tackling any of these items we may do them twenty times in our minds, getting a little tenser each time. Analysing the cause of this energy wastage, we will often find not that there is insufficient time, but that owing to lack of concentration and forethought we have frittered away both time and nerve-force. To control a restless mind is a task which can only be accomplished by steadily building an inner quietness and a

God-will. Star-breathing practised gently and persistently will gradually bring both will-power and clearer vision to the over-taxed mind and will strengthen the whole nervous system. It is our lifeline to our higher self.

Medical research has demonstrated the importance of the ductless glands in the functioning both of mind and body, and hormone extracts are now commonly prescribed for many conditions. Knowledge of the function of the ductless glands is far from modern: through many centuries, more particularly in the East, sages have stressed their significance, not only from the physical but also from the spiritual viewpoint. These glands are also linked with vital nerve-centres in the body which are fed by the bloodstream. With every breath the bloodstream is cleansed and recharged, not only with oxygen from the air but with divine life-force, if we will but take the trouble to feel this consciously, and allow the light to flow in. The more efficient and perfect our breathing technique, the better will the bloodstream be able to nourish the ductless glands which so radically affect all our activities and reactions.

The ductless glands are also connected with the psychic centres in the etheric body, those vortices of energy visible to a clairvoyant as dully glowing discs of light attached to the spinal column. They appear to be rather like flower buds at the end of a twining stalk, like that of the convolvulus. These energy centres are the connecting link between the soul and the physical body. They may also be described as the windows of the soul, through which the light can enter to purify and recharge our whole being.

This is how Star-breathing, affecting as it does the ductless glands and nervous system, can help us to draw upon a constant source of divine energy and strength. We all have within ourselves the power to change, to bring harmony into our lives and renewal to our bodies if we will make the effort to learn how to do so.

Humanity has reached a most important stage of evolution. The human mind is being quickened and inspired to solve many of the problems of the physical life, physical matter; but, which is even more important, man has reached the stage when he must learn the secret of consciously managing his own body, learning how to draw from the Cosmos the life-currents which will restore and renew the physical vehicle. We have to learn to live with the pressures of our civilisation. We have to learn how to bring our bodies under the quiet control of the spirit so that we can appreciate more fully the wonderful vistas of knowledge and creative expression which will open before us as our minds become more able to respond.

In order to breathe freely, so that the life-force can flow through all the different vehicles (physical, etheric, emotional and mental), it is important that the spine should be held as straight and erect as we can manage – not in any way stiffly, but as if the body was supported by a thread of light, rather like a strong piece of elastic coming down from a shining star above our heads and magically hooked onto the top of the head at the back.

To help you to get the feel of this, place the fingertips just beneath both ears. Now gently, with light pressure, slide them back along the base of the skull until the fingers meet, then slide the fingers up the back of the head so that the palms are gently cupping the head with the hair sliding through the fingers. Now gently close the fingers to grip the top hair and pull upwards, thinking of a line of light, a piece of elastic, which is drawing the top of your head upward. Hold this while you count ten, then let go of the hair and stand normally but consciously relaxing your shoulders down away from your ears, while still thinking of the pull of the elastic, which I always call my 'Star-hook'. It is a great help to think of the 'Star-hook' many times a day especially when life presses. The very thought of the line of light linking one with the shining Star of the real self is steadying, while the conscious relaxation of the shoulders and the stretching of the back of the neck helps to open up the chest so that the lungs can breathe more fully and freely. The double control will give a feeling of opening the heart-centre to the light. In old-fashioned words, 'We lift up our hearts unto the Lord'.

With these simple movements you will feel an unaccustomed sense of lightness and ease in your head, neck and shoulders, a release of tension. For a few moments think of the Sun–Star shining above you and let your breathing become quiet and even as you consciously enjoy the feeling of lightness and support from the heavens. To use one of Sir George Trevelyan's phrases, 'Let us learn to use the pull of levity (light) to counteract and balance the pull of gravity'.

Because of gravity, however, it is often easier to get the feel of a truly straight spine when lying flat on the floor than when we are standing or sitting. If you find it difficult to get down on the floor, you may like to have a piece of board cut, just long enough and wide enough for you to lie full length. This can be placed on the bed or across two chairs. The reason for using the hard floor or the board is that the rigid surface will not only support your spine, but help your muscles to become more accustomed to the straight position. You are putting yourself in what F. Matthias Alexander, the great exponent of improved posture for improved health, termed 'a position of mechanical advantage'!

Whether you use floor or board, cover it with a thick blanket so that your back does not feel chilled, and lie flat on your back with the top of your head resting on a book about two inches (50 cm) thick. Place it so that the back of your neck feels free and stretched. Slide your fingers up through your hair (as previously described for the 'Star-hook') and just rest the back of your head on the book so that the neck feels free and stretched, while your chin is gently drawn

29

down by gravity. You may need to experiment a little to find the thickness of book which is right for you – one which stretches the neck just a little so that it feels free and relaxed. Only the upper part of your head should be resting on the book, otherwise this will not happen.

If your back is at all stiff or painful do not attempt to lie with your legs stretched out. Have a chair or stool close up to your buttocks and rest your legs and feet on this so that your thighs form a right-angle with your trunk. This will rest your back and help you gradually to flatten it so that there is not such a pronounced curve in the lumbar region.

Now take your mind to your shoulders. Relax them down away from your ears and stretch out your arms comfortably at each side, palms uppermost. This position will again give

1   Resting the head. Slide your fingers through your hair *(above)* and then rest the back of your head on the book

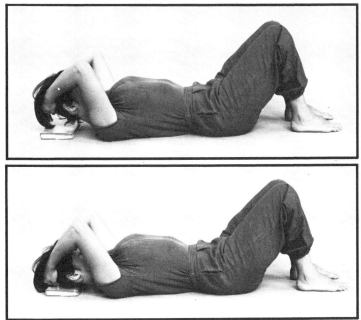

you a feeling of opening up chest and heart to the light and you can let all tension slip away from the shoulders and back of the neck. All of us collect much tension here, especially where the neck joins the shoulders. A natural reaction to strain is to tense the shoulders and to walk about with them hunched, and with the chin poking forward as if we have to take life's blows on the chin!

Let all this tension go. Relax the shoulders down, feel the stretch of the back of your neck and the Star-hook linking you to the world of light, and just quietly listen to your breathing.

Imagine above you a beautiful shining Star. See its rays pouring down – like a wigwam of light, protecting and enfolding you with divine light and energy. In your mind, talk to your neck and shoulders. Tell them to relax, to allow full inflow of the shining life-force into your lungs, so that it can permeate the bloodstream and then soothe and heal every cell of your being. Really concentrate for a minute or two on these affirmations, enjoying the stretch of your neck and the peace of your quiet, slow breathing. Now think of your head gently swivelling to the right as far as it can go (neck stretched – chin in). *Don't do it – think it*; then relax and let it happen. The book will help you to keep the neck stretched and relaxed as you turn your head. Rest for at least a minute in this position, quietly breathing in the Light. If you feel any muscular strain or ache in shoulder or neck, tell the muscles to relax more – to let go – let go – let go. Mentally draw the light to them, gently breathing it in and directing it. Now think of the head slowly swivelling back and round as far as it will go in the opposite direction. *Don't do it, think it* clearly, then relax and let it happen. Again rest and in your mind talk to the muscles telling them to relax as you breathe in the light, directing it to any little aches and tensions. Open your whole being to the healing light which is being drawn into your body with every breath. Now bring your head back to the centre and rest quietly, listening to your breathing. Feel the flow of light into your heart. Picture the bloodstream recharged with life and energy radiating through every cell of your body bringing strength, health, rejuvenation.

This position, lying flat on the back, is known to yoga students as *savasana* or the 'corpse' posture. It expresses physically the complete surrender of the little everyday self to the healing strength of the divine self. To lie in this position for ten minutes of quiet Star-breathing is a most restoring exercise which can help one to cope with the busiest day without undue strain. The important thing is to try to arrange to break off activity before you become too tired. It will charge your batteries and help you to review your problems in true perspective. If you can manage to

2 *Savasana*, the 'corpse' posture. If your back is stiff or painful use the stool to help you gradually flatten any curve in the lumbar region

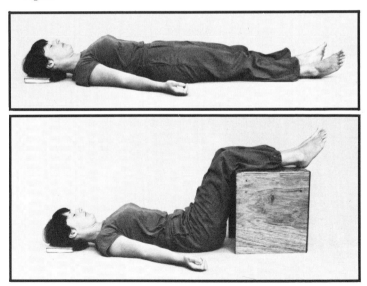

practise this relaxation and Star-breathing two or three times during the course of a day you will find yourself gradually much calmer and more in command.

During one of your times on the floor each day you should try to practise three simple movements which will help you to build into your body-mind or body-elemental a conscious awareness of the feel of the correct posture, so that this will affect your ordinary, everyday movements. Good posture is a relaxed posture with all the different sets of muscles involved balancing each other perfectly. To keep these muscles in a state of tonicity need not involve vigorous exercises. The simple daily movements of walking, standing, sitting and breathing, correctly performed, will provide the body with sufficient exercise to keep it healthy and flexible throughout a long life. The trouble is that such is our life-style, particularly in the West, that we have lost the feeling for correct posture. Our bodies, responding to the pull of gravity, have formed a habit of slumping down which feels normal and right. This slump involves strain and tension in some muscles and too much slackness in others, so that the uneven balance causes strain. Because this has become habitual we are unaware of the lack of balance, except for the warning of little muscular aches and pains which become accentuated as we grow older. The difficulty everyone faces when trying to improve posture is that the old habits are so strong that it takes a certain amount of wiliness to replace them with better ones. The three movements which should help are those which now follow.

First Movement

Lying peacefully in the savasana position, take your mind again to the alignment of your head and shoulders. Is the back of your neck comfortably free and stretched? Is your chin sinking towards your throat and are your shoulders relaxing down, away from your ears? See and feel the ideal poise of the head; visualise the clear straight channel from the top of the head down the neck and spine to the heart centre. Breathe slowly and peacefully. Now as you breathe out, relax and open your jaw in a whispered vowel sound – 'aaah' – or 'ooo', 'ay', 'aw', 'ee', if you prefer. Just one vowel sound, but whisper it right to the very end of the breath; and then wait with jaw still relaxed for a slow count of ten. Then close your mouth and breathe quietly again, enjoying the beautifully relaxed position of the head with the back of the neck stretched and the chin in. Repeat this three or four more times, each time expelling every vestige of breath and letting the jaw relax open as you count ten. You may well find yourself giving a deeply satisfying yawn, which will help to loosen up the chest and relax the intercostal muscles so that your breathing becomes automatically deep. Don't force anything – just relax and let it happen and peacefully continue your 'Star-breathing'.

This is one of the recommendations in F. Matthias Alexander's book *Man's Supreme Inheritance* (Methuen, 1910). He says, 'The quantity of residual air in the lungs is greatly increased, and if the expired air is always converted into a controlled whispered vowel during the practice of the breathing exercises very great benefits accrue, notably those derived from the prolonged duration of air in the lungs, and the proper inter-thoracic pressure necessary to force the adequate supply of oxygen into the blood and eliminate the due quantity of CO_2.

'The employment of these whispered tones means the proper use of the vocal organs in a form of vocalisation little associated with ordinary bad habits, and that perfect co-ordination of the parts concerned which is inseparable from adequately controlled whisper vocalisation.

'There is a rapid clearing of the skin, the white face becoming a natural colour, and a reduction of fat in the obese by its being burnt off with the extra oxygen supply.'

34

This first exercise is important, because if it is performed without fail every day, preferably first thing in the morning or at night before sleeping, the feeling for the correct poise of the head will grow in your subconscious mind. Many times during the day you will find yourself automatically stretching the back of your neck, relaxing your shoulders down and thinking of the beautiful line of light shining down into your heart from the blazing Star above your head. This Star, the symbol of the higher self, the real shining self which lives constantly in the heavens, will heal and strengthen you; will help you to keep calm and poised in all trying circumstances.

Second Movement

Lie on your back with head and shoulders aligned as before (think the directions: 'Star-hook' – neck free and stretched – chin in – shoulders relaxed down away from the ears). Breathe slowly and peacefully. If your legs are stretched out, visualise bending your knees and drawing your feet up towards your buttocks – feet flat on the floor about 15 inches apart. *Don't do it – think it.* Then relax and let it happen. If your legs are up on a chair or stool you can do the movement from there. Can you feel the whole length of your spine lying along the floor, or is there a gap at the waistline? If so, visualise the spine flat against the floor; but if this is at all difficult, leave it for the present. Don't try to *do* it. It will right itself eventually without conscious muscular effort. The small movements that you practise each day combined with the steady thought of the correct position will gradually bring your body into beautiful alignment, but you must be patient and persistent. Keep on every day regularly with these small movements, remembering that the most important thing of all is the direction of the light, the life-force, through visualisation and then relaxation. You will be surprised at the increasing sense of freedom and poise which comes to your body.

Focus your vision just between your knees – which is easy if your head is poised correctly with back of neck stretched and free. Give the mental directions: 'Lift the base of the spine, the coccyx area, off the floor by a gentle tightening of the muscles in the groin.' Do not do this yet; just think about it. Picture the movement. See the light flowing down the spine, then drawing up the muscles in the groin to lift the very lowest part of the spine, the coccyx area, a little off the floor. Give the mental direction, then relax and let it happen. Hold the position for a slow count of ten. Relax and repeat, not just the movement but the whole process. You

3   Lifting the coccyx off the floor (notice the changed angle of the pelvis)

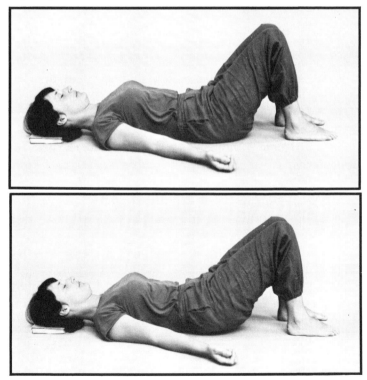

will find it easier if you breathe in as you picture the movement, and then let the groin muscles perform the lifting action as you exhale. Remember that the movement itself is not as important as the thinking about it, mentally giving the direction and then surrendering to the light, the life-force. It is this conscious uniting of the body of light with the physical body that is going to produce the result. After lifting the coccyx four or five times from the floor in this way, relax, straighten the legs if you were lying flat, and gently continue the Star-breathing; visualising the Light flowing right down your straight spine, flowing along all the nerve channels, and revitalising your whole being. Regular practice of these beautiful, peaceful routines will help you not only to straighten your spine and bring your body back into balance but will give you a calm attitude towards the little strains of life. You will find yourself taking them much more philo-sophically, 'in your stride', when you hold the contact with the beautiful Star of your real self.

Third Movement

The last of the movements performed in a lying-down position is a splendid preparation for the type of deep-breathing which is the basis of buoyant health. Most of us pay little attention to our breathing during everyday life. We take it for granted and only become aware of it in vigorous exercise, or if some soreness or inflammation obstructs the breathing passages. Yet it is the one key function of the body over which we have a certain amount of conscious control. The heart pumps and the blood circulates without our knowing anything about it. The digestive and genital systems function according to their own rhythm and beyond our volition, but breathing we can to some extent regulate. Herein lies an important key to man's conscious control of other aspects of his being: his nervous and emotional reactions and later on his soul-development.

People normally take rather shallow breaths unless some strenuous exercise forces them to breathe deeply to re-oxygenate the body. The expression, 'I am out of breath', indicates that our need for oxygen is forcing the chest muscles and the diaphragm to work harder to draw in fresh air. Although the body can exist placidly with habitual shallow breathing, it is amazing how much more energy and vitality can be released and enjoyed if we can form a spontaneous habit of expanding the lower ribs, so that with every breath we fill the lower as well as the upper part of the lungs. There is no doubt that relaxed lower-lung breathing, especially if combined with a conscious drawing-in of the divine light, can restore health and energy to a limp, depleted body. This natural, deep breathing can become much easier and indeed habitual by regular practice of this third exercise.

You are lying on your blanket on the floor or board, with the book supporting the back of your head, so that the neck is gently stretched and gravity is drawing your head and chin into the correct position; your spine is as relaxed and flat as possible, your feet apart (about fifteen to eighteen inches). You feel very peaceful and easy. Your shoulders are comfortably relaxed down, away from your ears with arms and hands on the floor, palms upward, about nine inches away from your body.

Visualise the shining Star of your real self, its light pouring upon you, finding a free passage through the top of your head and down the spine, filling the heart and the whole nervous system with light, with every gentle breath you take.

Now if you feel along your rib-cage, from the central breastbone right down to the sides, you will find that the lowest part moves with every breath you take, or it should do. With shallow breathing it hardly moves at all. You will be taking easy little breaths at the top of your chest; or if you are a man, it will probably be the abdomen which moves. In the deeper breathing which is our aim, the lower ribs will swing out, allowing the diaphragm (the umbrella-shaped muscle which divides the chest from the abdomen) to flatten so that the lower parts of the lungs – which are much more capacious than the upper parts – can be filled with fresh air. In this exercise, which like the other two should be performed each morning (and/or evening) for the rest of your life, we are not concentrating upon the breathing itself, but the means whereby those lower ribs can become more flexible and active.

Lying flat and relaxed on your board (or floor) place your palms on the lower ribs and mentally give the direction, 'Let the lower ribs expand'. Visualise the lower ribs widening to make more space in the chest. Now relax and let it happen. At first you may feel very little, just the slightest movement, but persevere. Again give the direction, 'Let the lower ribs expand'; visualise it if you can, then let it happen. You may feel a little more movement this time, but do not feel worried if there is only slight response. Persevere for about five times just giving the direction, 'Let the lower ribs expand', visualising, relaxing, and then letting the life-force do it.

If you feel an appreciable movement after one or two tries, hold the muscular contraction for a second or two and take a tiny breath, through the nose, thinking it in that lower region of your lungs. Speakers and singers who have been trained in diaphragmatic breathing will understand this perfectly, but for many people it will be a new experience to become aware of breathing in this region. We would emphasise that this is not in itself a breathing exercise. Do not attempt to make it so. It is just the regular performance, with thought and understanding, of a tiny movement which will eventually become so automatic that it happens quite unconsciously; but it is a key to that easy, deep diaphragmatic breathing which when it becomes part of our daily living will bring the joy of increased vitality and poise. The little breath which you take at the end of the movement of the ribs is almost automatic. It will help you to realise how this rib movement can lead to the habit of good, deep breathing.

These simple movements, lying on board or floor, should become a pleasurable part of the daily routine. The whole group of movements can be peacefully completed within ten minutes, and could even form part of a morning or evening meditation. To regard them in this way will bring much more satisfactory results than to think of them as a chore to be performed, 'a daily dozen', which is just what they are not. Performed correctly, when you concentrate not on the movements themselves but on the inflow of the life-force into the body, they bring an increasing sense of peace and relaxation; a confidence in the power of the Great White Spirit within and around us to bring the physical body to a state of wholeness and beauty.

People who find some difficulty in regular meditation may respond to this routine, for the physical body is a creature of habit. Once it has become accustomed to act in a certain way it will want to continue. Since mental and spiritual attunement is an important feature of the practice, this too will become much more automatic. You may even find yourself really *wanting* to start earlier to make time for a longer period of quiet aspiration when the exercises are finished.

There is no doubt that you will in time be pleased and surprised to notice how your daily practice of these small movements is building into the subconscious mind an awareness of how the body should feel when it is perfectly poised; no muscular strain anywhere, but a lovely feeling of spring and lightness which is due to the perfect polarisation of the body with the heart-centre – the source of life. It is constantly energised and revitalised through easy deep-breathing, which in turn leads to a more peaceful and relaxed mental state.

4

EXERCISE WITHOUT EXERCISES

MOST PEOPLE ARE well aware of the body's need for exercise, but apart from sports enthusiasts and those who for professional reasons must keep a lithe figure, few have the energy or will-power to perform a 'daily dozen'. This is probably just as well, for the enthusiastic amateur, too vigorously jerking unaccustomed muscles, can easily cause himself damage through strain. This particularly applies to the traditional toe-touching exercises which can result in persistent trouble in the lower back.

Nevertheless, exercise is a real health need, which with a little knowledge and perseverance can be adequately met during the normal day's activities. The human body is a most wonderfully constructed organism, demonstrating in all its functions the same law of balance which manifests throughout the universe. The process of digestion takes place through the balancing interaction of acid and alkaline secretions in mouth, stomach and intestines. Breathing involves a constant interchange of gases in the lungs, thus cleansing and vitalising the bloodstream. Every physical movement is the result of contracting and relaxing perfectly balanced sets of muscles; and the *correct* performance of the four basic actions of breathing, sitting, standing and walking can give the body continuous and perfect exercise, for the alternate stretching and contraction involved in the ordinary movements gently exercises the muscles all the time.

Most people's daily work entails some form of continuous muscular strain. If the work is of a sedentary, clerical type, there will be a tendency to strain and tension at the back of the neck and in the shoulder and arm used for writing. This tension, combined with carrying heavy loads of textbooks, often causes schoolchildren and students to adopt a posture with one shoulder habitually higher than the other. Unless this is observed and corrected, it can lead to a lifetime of small muscular discomforts as the body settles itself into one-sidedness. Constant lifting, or one-sided movement of any kind will cause a gradual tendency to a lop-sided posture; even the smallest movement constantly performed will gradually make its mark in the physical stance, so that it is often quite easy to guess their type of occupation from a person's general bearing.

Is *your* daily work spoiling your posture and causing minor aches and pains through lack of balance? Stand unclad before a long mirror in your normal upright posture and imagine a plumb-line, dropped from the centre of your brow to your toes. This should lie exactly in front of the hollow in the throat, the centre of the breastbone, and the navel, and fall between the feet. On either side of this straight line, the shoulders, the nipples and the hip-bones should be symmetrically balanced. If you are a sedentary worker, or are accustomed to carrying heavy bags on one side of the body (even a heavy handbag can do it) the chances are that you will notice one shoulder, one nipple and one hip higher than the other, and the whole body may have a slight twist. If this is the case, you can start your rehabilitation by becoming aware of the way you perform all your regular actions such as cleaning teeth, shaving, putting on make-up, brushing hair, unscrewing bottle-tops, turning on taps and all the many small actions of everyday life, including of course writing. You may well be surprised at how much more one hand works than the other. It is not difficult, once you are aware of the imbalance, to remember to use the opposite hand until gradually you are much more ambidextrous, and until the subconscious twist of the posture begins to straighten.

Also to help restore the balance, you could try to fit a few gentle stretching and swinging movements into your daily routine. Notice which side droops, and as often as you can remember stretch up as high as you can on that side, as if you are reaching for a tempting fruit. Stretch both hands above your head, but reach out higher and more frequently from the side that droops. Do this many times each day, or whenever you feel a little weary and stiff, and then swing your arms loosely over your head and round in large circular movements to relax the shoulders. Before going to sleep at night, and first thing in the morning, stretch out firmly but gently in bed. With the legs pressed down against the mattress and toes turned up stretch first one heel then the other towards the bottom of the bed, with particular attention to the drooping side. Alternately stretch the arms above the head in the same way, paying special attention to the unbalanced side.

You will probably not find it difficult to trace the imbalance either to some habitual action in your work or to some unconscious postural habit, such as standing with your weight on one foot: little actions in themselves but, constantly performed, they are like the constant drip of water which wears away a stone, or builds a stalagmite. Once you become aware of the cause of the trouble, you can watch for the bad habit and keep trying to restore the balance and release the tension. If you find yourself writing with tense hand, shoulder and neck, frequently put down your pen, stretch your arms and do a few neck and head turning exercises. Such exercise as this is not tiresome or energy-consuming, for in restoring the balance it brings a certain pleasure and feeling of relaxation. If you habitually carry a handbag or briefcase in one hand, remember to change hands frequently and in your work train yourself to be a little more ambidextrous.

A straight but flexible spine plays a large part in physical and mental well-being. Once we become fully conscious of this, we will no longer loll in armchairs or use any available prop to support us when we must stand. Bad postures which seem comfortable through habitual use, far from being restful and relaxing, actually strain certain organs and muscles, whilst allowing others to become flabby and gummed up with fatty tissue. This causes the body to lose its vigour and beauty and leads it to develop increased girth in the waist and abdomen, while drooping shoulders and sunken chest indicate muscular stiffness and inflexibility which greatly decrease the air capacity in the lungs.

The body is so perfectly constructed that if we can train ourselves to make all the little movements required in daily living as easily and perfectly as nature intended, many of the muscles will be kept in a perfect state of tonicity and health. This, however, is easier said than done, because the weight of the head, unless it is perfectly poised on the neck and spine, tends to drag the whole body forward and downward. You can feel this for yourself. Imagine the line of light, the piece of elastic coming down from the Star, hooked on to the back of your head pulling you up gently but firmly so that the chin is drawn in. Let the shoulders relax down away from the ears and think of opening up your heart to the light which is pouring down from the Star. You will feel a sense of lightness and ease about the head and shoulders as if a weight had slipped off. Through the stretch of the back of the neck and the head you feel the whole body gently pulled into alignment. Now imagine that the elastic has been cut and you slump. The chin will jut forward and immediately the weight of the head will pull you into a round-shouldered position. You will feel the pull of gravity. The whole body will feel heavier, and obviously it will tire more quickly – all because the weight of the head is not properly poised at the top of the straight spine with the back of the neck freely stretched.

Most people spend their time performing tasks which encourage them to slump. From an early age most children are expected to work bent over their desks, while the shape of modern easy chairs and car seats, comfortable and well-upholstered though they seem, does not help. Faulty posture becomes so customary that it feels right. To stretch up and hold the body erect feels unnatural. It apparently imposes strain upon unaccustomed muscles, and is such an effort that most people soon give up. This is why the technique of practising regularly the small adjustments of the body needed to improve posture, combined with the power of auto-suggestion, can be so helpful. From the beginning, when talking to his students about the importance of the straight spine both for health and for spiritual unfoldment, White Eagle emphasised that it was a question more of the mind than the body. He explained that the body-elemental feels a natural pull downward towards the earth but the spirit of man, the higher consciousness, can direct and train the body-elemental even as a wise master will train a pet animal.

Man is not yet aware of the wonderful controlling influence which the higher mind can exert on the body-elemental. It is simple but not easy because it requires considerable effort and perseverance. The body-elemental is a creature of instinct, reacting immediately and spontaneously to its feelings and sensations. In the animal world, particularly with animals in their natural state, this instinctive reaction to primitive feelings is a help and protection since the animal is guided and directed by the group soul watching over that particular species.

With the development of his mental powers, and his achievement of civilisation and culture, man outgrows the direction and protection of the animal group soul. He has become increasingly individualised, learning to live by mind and reason, learning to understand and adjust to the laws of life and growth. Because civilised life is so different from that of primitive communities, man has to take increasing personal control and responsibility for managing his physical mechanism so that it will adjust easily and healthfully to the situation in which he finds himself. We cannot return to primitive conditions. The whole of mankind is now evolving to a new state of consciousness, new ways of living. It is possible for everyone who gives their mind to it to learn how to adjust their body to the new conditions, but each person does it for himself, and must keep in mind the goal he wants to achieve. Quietly, steadily, purposefully, he must train the body in the small movements which will gradually give an awareness of the 'feel' of good posture in any circumstances.

Standing Straight

To get the 'feel' of the correct standing posture, find a door or wall that has no wainscoting or protuberance to break the flat surface. With feet about twelve inches apart (no shoes) stand with your heels, buttocks and shoulders touching the wall. The back of your head may easily touch the wall, but if not, in no way strain to make it do so. Visualise the Star shining above your head and the straight line of light, your piece of elastic, hooked on to the top of your head at the back. Hands and arms should hang loosely at your sides while your eyes look straight ahead. Make sure that the shoulders are relaxed. Tell them to relax down, down, down and watch the body-elemental obeying. Try to become conscious of how your own little animal, the body-elemental, the horse on which you ride, happily obeys your firm instruction if you will allow it to do so.

Imagine that you have quite a heavy tail hanging from the base of your spine. It is like a weight pulling your coccyx down, even as the 'Star-hook' is pulling the top of your head up so that there is a gentle feeling of stretch to the whole spine. Now imagine that this heavy tail is coming forward

46

through your legs, pulling your coccyx even more under you. You may like to bend your knees to get the feel of this 'tail' being tucked in. You are now going to keep the thought of that gently stretched spine, tail tucked in, as you rise onto your toes. Just think about it, imagine it first, then let the body obey your thought. 'Relax and let it happen.' The wall will be a reminder of that line of light which is pulling you upwards, even as the heavy tail is pulling the coccyx under and adjusting the position of the pelvis. Repeat this movement four or five times, standing against the wall, each

4   Standing straight. *Left:* the basic position. *Centre:* bending the knees to get the feel of the 'tail' being tucked in. *Right:* rising onto the toes

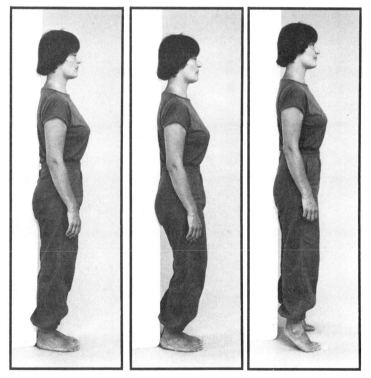

time imagining the action first and then relaxing fully to the pull of the line of light from that beautiful Star, your higher self, which is taking control of the physical atoms of the body.

Now walk away from the wall, trying to keep the feeling of the body supported by your 'Star-hook', with shoulders loose and relaxed, chest and heart open to the light, and the tail pulled down and under. Try to repeat this exercise several times during the day whenever the opportunity arises. When you feel quite happy with this movement, probably after you have been doing it for two or three weeks, you can add a further development. As you rise onto your toes and bring your 'tail' under, think of the arms being raised and stretched forward at shoulder level, as if you were trying to touch the opposite wall, but again with shoulders down and arms beautifully relaxed. Think it, direct the body-elemental, and relax into the position. Repeat this a few times with your back against the wall, then walk forward, feeling your line of light strengthening and upholding you.

This will help you gradually to strengthen the muscles in the groin so that the lumbar curve is less emphasised; and in time as you stand against the wall you will only just be able to pass your flattened hand between the wall and the curve of the waist. But don't try to force this or you will immediately become tense and block the flow of the life-force. Just quietly continue to give mental directions for the small easy movements, and let the body-elemental obey.

The final routine in this standing group is standing on one leg. You may be able to do this quite easily without losing your balance but, just in case, stand fairly close to a wall so that you can touch it to support yourself. Think your usual instructions. Feel the line of light, the 'Star-hook', which is drawing your head into the correct position; feel the shoulders relaxing down, down, down and the heart open to the light. Now think of one leg lifted at right angles, bent at the knee with the foot hanging loosely and comfortably. Unless you are very stiff the toe will automatically be pointing down. The spine is stretched, yet relaxed, and your whole body easily poised on the one leg. Think through the whole exercise first but do not do it. Now relax, think of the shining Star above your head and let the light flow through you to produce the required result. Hold the position for a few seconds, then let the foot return to the floor, the ball of the foot taking the weight first. Repeat the process with the other foot. Lift each knee about five times.

This sounds a simple and possibly boring movement, but it is surprising how fascinating the exercise becomes when you apply the directing, visualising and relaxing process. You begin to learn a great deal about your body and its response to thought, also about your own powers of concentration.

As you become more confident in this exercise, see if you can do it with your eyes shut. You will have quite a surprise! It is much more difficult than it sounds, but the thought of that Star, shining steadily above your head, will eventually keep you perfectly poised standing on one leg with your eyes closed; but it will take time and patience. The whole object of the exercise is to help you to realise how the thought of the body beautifully poised under the Star will give you steady balance and a feeling of peace.

It is a good idea to do this balancing exercise before going to bed, especially if your mind is a little overwrought with the affairs of the day. When you have reached the stage of trying to do it with your eyes closed, you will realise that it is impossible unless you focus your mind on the Star, or some other object which gives you a feeling of steady strength. This routine will help you to quieten down the tensions of your day and find that beautiful balance or union of the lower with the higher self, symbolised by the Star.

Constant repetition of thought direction into these small movements is an essential part of success in harnessing the power of the body-elemental. In order to make these directions fully effective we must keep experiencing the 'feel' of the correct posture of head, neck, shoulders and back. This is why the lying-down movements are so helpful and why it is a good idea to create for ourselves a little formula of directions which we repeat, if possible, in a whispered command to the body-elemental many times a day, so that gradually a new good habit ousts the old bad one.

We must make the effort ourselves: feel and think each movement through for ourselves. Nobody else can do it for us. Reading and study of countless books won't help – in fact this could leave us more confused. We must learn ourselves the 'feel' of each movement and come thoroughly to understand our own bodies, then formulate in our own way the routine instructions which will become for us a mantram for constant repetition.

My own directions have evolved as follows. They help me to remember to practise the small movements many times a day so that these are gradually becoming habitual. You will probably evolve something entirely different. No matter, so long as you think them through, experience their effect and use the same formula each time, for the body-elemental responds to childlike repetition.

If it is not convenient to pull up the hair at the top of my head, I picture it, and clearly *think* the feeling. I picture the Star shining down, and from it a piece of elastic with a little hook at the end, which hooks on to the top of my head so that the line of light is established. All this formulates into the words 'Star-hook'. This gives me the feeling of a beautifully free stretch at the back of the neck, specially where it joins the shoulders, with head poised forwards and the chin falling inwards.

The next direction is 'Relax shoulders, *down, down, down*'

(I emphasise this because I notice that at the first sign of stress they hunch up round my ears!). Then follows 'Let the heart and chest be open to the light', and I picture the heart opening like a flower to absorb the warmth, strength and healing of the Sun–Star.

Finally comes the instruction 'Bring tail down and under'.

These directions are shortened into a quick personal formula:

1. Star-hook
2. Shoulders down, down, down
3. Heart lifted to light
4. Tail down and under.

Maybe these ideas will help you to formulate your own mantram of directions.

Sitting Straight

Since many people have to spend much of their time sitting at their work, this position will be the one in which they can take most of their exercise. Unless they consciously train themselves in correct posture they will lay the foundations of innumerable aches and pains due to the wrong use of the body mechanisms. Chairs nearly always have their backs at the wrong angle, so that it is impossible to use their support if you are making an effort to sit upright. Indeed, a stool of the correct height and with a firmly padded seat can be far more helpful and comfortable than many chairs, even those which are specially made to support backs. Strictly speaking, if the spine is upright with the head properly balanced, it should not need support. The correct sitting position is so comfortable and easy and the body is so well balanced that one should be able to remain in this position for a long time without strain.

In the East, where so many people are accustomed to sitting on the floor, the straight spine of the yogi is much more of a norm. It is a vital health secret, for when the spine is held upright with the back of the neck freely stretched, head poised, shoulders relaxed and heart raised ('Star-hook'), breathing automatically becomes deeper; digestion is improved, as well as all the other internal functions. In the upright sitting position the muscles are all co-ordinating in the way nature intended, and once the position has become habitual there will be far less tendency to the little aches and strains in back, shoulders and neck, from which so many people suffer.

Because of the habitual misuse of our muscles the upright position may at first feel stiff and unnatural, and if we force ourselves into it, we will soon give up the attempt because of the strain and discomfort. This is why we so strongly recommend constantly and patiently *thinking* the right posture and practising at odd times throughout the day the small movements which will eventually become so automatic that they lead us easily into maintaining it.

In practising the small movements which lead to good sitting and to rising easily from the sitting position, it is helpful first to find the right chair. This should have a firm seat and an upright back, but more especially it should be of a height which enables the feet to be placed comfortably on the floor, the legs forming a right angle at the knee and the straight spine forming a right angle with the thigh. Once you find the right chair (or stool), it is a good idea to use it constantly in your normal daily activities so that the very feel of the chair will bring into your mind the mental direction that you are constantly giving to your body. To adjust the height of your chair or stool, you may need to use a flat, firm cushion or to place your feet on a board or cork bathmat. It is worth experimenting until you find exactly the right and comfortable position, because only then will the body get the 'feel' of the true balance.

Now, sit down comfortably and imagine your spine as

straight as it is when you are standing up against the wall. Think your own directions. You will probably find it helpful to adjust the poise of your head with the hands (hair-pulling!); to feel your 'Star-hook'; and then be sure to relax the shoulders, lift and open the heart, and for a few moments enjoy the beautifully free, straight upright posture. This is what we are hoping eventually to maintain all the time. Think it – relax into it – and enjoy the feeling of the life-force flowing freely down the gently stretched spine as you peacefully breathe in the light. Feel the air flowing deep into the lungs filling the heart with light, then radiate that light out into the world.

The object of the next exercise is so to loosen and straighten the pelvic muscles that you will be able to sit down and get up from the chair gracefully, without the help of the hands. Place the feet flat on the floor, a little apart, and *let the knees spread comfortably*. This is important. Rest the forearms, palms upwards, comfortably along the thighs to assist your keeping a straight back as you bend forward. Now, take your thoughts to the very base of the spine. Think of leaning forward from this point, with the spine absolutely straight – back of the neck freely stretched ('Star-hook'), shoulders relaxed. Think through the points clearly. Now let it happen. You will go forward so easily and lightly, spine absolutely straight. Rest a moment, then think through coming up again. Think your directions and relax into it.

Pause for a few moments, feel the shining Star above your head, and once more breathe quietly enjoying the feeling of the life-force flowing down your straight, relaxed spine. Again think through the movements, then relax into the forward bend, keeping the spine straight. You will probably go a little bit further this time, but don't strain. Think from the bottom of the spine and be sure to keep the whole line straight. Keep your 'Star-hook' well attached, neck freely stretched and shoulders down. This sounds an easy movement but if it is possible for you to watch yourself in a mirror you will quite likely notice a strong tendency to curl forward at the waist and for the chin to jut forward. So be sure to focus your attention on stretching the back of the neck and move from the very base of the spine, because thinking of those two points will help you get the picture of the long, straight line the spine should form. The whole movement is rather like the opening and shutting of a penknife. Perhaps the opening and shutting of a pair of compasses might be an even better simile, because there is no spring in the compasses – just the smooth opening and shutting at the joint. Remind yourself frequently that it is the hip, the very base of the spine, that is being loosened and made more flexible. Gently, perform the movement several times, swinging backwards and forwards thinking of your beautifully straight spine and flexible hip-joint. Always think the movement through first and never strain to make yourself go further than your hips will allow. Otherwise you will defeat your own object, and probably curl at the waist. In all these small movements never rush into action. *Always* think first (visualising if you can the straight spine with the light flowing through the top of the head right down to the base – the hip-joint). Then relax and enjoy the physical sensation.

When you find this exercise easy and pleasant and are sure that you are keeping your back straight as you swing forward, you can use the movement for rising from your chair. Do this bending exercise two or three times, working up a momentum. Keep thinking your special directions, then see yourself rising easily from the chair and straightening up. Now relax and let the life-force carry you into the stand-up position. Pause for a moment, thinking still of the straight, stretched spine with the beautiful flow of the life-force from the crown of the head down the spine and right down the legs to the feet. Now, with the backs of your legs touching the chair, think again this penknife movement, and

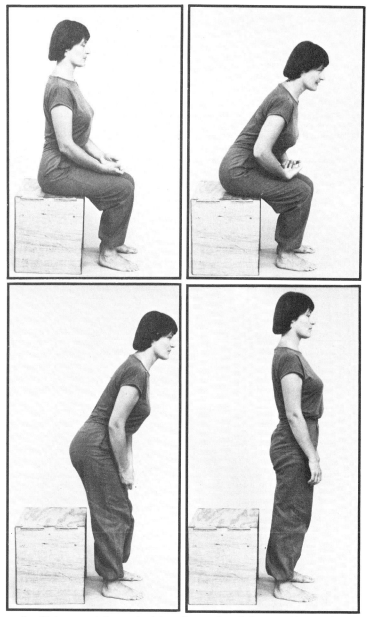

5 Sitting straight and rising from the sitting position. The sequence of photographs shows how natural the rising motion is when the thought is directed properly

55

relax back into the sitting position with no help from your hands.

It will be quite a long time before these two movements of standing and sitting without the help of your hands and keeping your spine absolutely straight become automatic, for the habit of sitting badly, jutting the chin and curling up the spine as you struggle out of the chair, is probably deeply ingrained. This is why once you have started to practise, it is a good idea to keep to the same chair which is correctly adjusted for you. The feel of your hard chair will remind you to keep thinking yourself into the right posture. Once you have started to practise the correct standing and sitting, do try very hard to stop and start again each time you find yourself doing it the wrong way, because each time you go back to your old way you will be helping to maintain the old, bad habit. Remember, you are trying to form a new good habit of use, and this is an important and crucial stage in your training. At the same time don't so worry about it that you become tense and stiff as you are practising. Remember the importance of the attunement to the Star, and from the higher self give your directions gently and firmly to the body-elemental. Practise the penknife or compass movement many times during the day and use the movement to get up from your chair. Practise rising and sitting properly as often as you can, and most of all, avoid sprawling in an easy chair. Try to remember to choose always a hard one, and if possible one of the correct height for you, for this will be a reminder.

Once this feeling for straight sitting and graceful rising from a chair has become established in your subconscious you will have reached an important stage in your progress. If you give your mind to the various activities you perform sitting down, you will soon become aware of those which present the greatest temptation to slump. For instance, in reading, you should try to adjust the position of your book so that you are sitting upright and are not tempted to curl forward from the waist with chin jutting out.

It is the cultivation of an awareness of what your body is doing that will help you gradually to replace the bad old habits with new good ones. This especially applies to the sitting position, and it is well worth while to think through all the daily routine to see how the position of your work can be adjusted so that you can constantly maintain that easy, straight spinal posture with the head poised – back of neck freely stretched, shoulders relaxed down, and heart-centre raised and open to the light. Think often of this posture. See the Star shining above your head and become aware of how the flow of that beautiful life-force is hindered whenever you slump and hold the head wrongly. This is the greatest possible incentive to maintaining the right position, because the feeling of peace and strength which flows into the body when it is held correctly has to be experienced to be believed. It is worth the continual practice of the small movements. Remember also that the sure foundation of correct posture lies in the constant regular performance of those three original exercises which you perform lying down and with your head resting on a book. These should never become a chore but form a harmonious part of the daily routine. They are almost a meditation in themselves, and will quicken the awareness of the body as a temple of the spirit; for each time they are performed they bring us under the ray of the beautiful, shining Star of the true self which will bring health, strength and renewal to the body.

5

'PUTTING YOUR BEST FOOT FORWARD'

WHEN THE FEET are painful or uncomfortable, we quickly become tired, tense and irritable. Irritability sparks off the same reaction in the people we contact, which they in turn vent on someone else until the effects of one pair of uncomfortable feet spread like ripples on the water after a stone has been thrown into a pond. Body, soul and mind are not separate entities and such close interconnection exists between them that unless every part is functioning correctly, the whole being is soon thrown out of harmony – and lack of harmony spells disease.

Compare our mental outlook when we are well fed, warm and comfortable, with when we are hungry, cold and in pain. It takes a well-poised and philosophical soul to remain tranquil in such circumstances, and oh, what trivial things can affect both bodily comfort and mental attitude!

Particularly is this true of the feet – the understandings. This is no meaningless pun, for the feet are closely allied to man's understanding. Pisces, which astrologically governs the feet, is ruled by Jupiter, the planet concerned with man's understanding of spiritual truth; and Pisces, a sign of the element Water, is connected with the soul or psyche. When Jesus washed the disciples' feet, and Peter, in his enthusiasm, asked for his hands and head to be cleansed as well, Jesus told him that if his feet were washed, his whole desire-nature would be purified. The sign of Pisces rules places and conditions of imprisonment and confinement. What is more restricting to the aspiring soul than painful or immobile feet? Yet, those who suffer chronically in this way will perhaps take comfort from the thought that during this incarnation their difficulties with the feet may be the means of cleansing the desire-nature and bringing to the soul that childlike simplicity and purity which will enable it to understand and recognise spiritual truth.

Through the feet we contact the magnetism of mother earth. They are the foundation of human poise and balance, and when kept in a healthy, flexible state they help in bringing peace and understanding to the mind. When the muscles of the feet are functioning perfectly we should be able to be quite unconscious of them from morning to night. Like the hands, they should be the servants of the higher self, carrying the body on its missions with grace and speed.

Unfortunately in the so-called civilised countries we have grown so far away from nature that it is rare to see beautiful feet except in young children. Fashion regularly decrees that shoes must possess a built-up heel, particularly for women, and many people regard high-heeled shoes as attractive and even essential to feminine charm. Yet the perfect functioning of the human body depends upon proper balance and co-ordination. Every muscle, every body chemical, is counterbalanced by its opposite, and all the life-processes are governed by the same rhythmic law. The feet control the fulcrum of the whole body.

Standing barefoot, with the weight evenly spread over the whole foot and a feeling of spring in the instep, with head and neck properly adjusted ('Star-hook' – shoulders relaxed – heart lifted – tail down under) we have perfect physical poise. If we raise the heels from the ground by our own effort, the centre of balance is slightly altered, but the poise of the body is maintained. But if we artificially raise the heels on supports, the correct balance of the body is immediately disturbed, the weight being automatically thrown on to the heels. To maintain the balance the knees have to be slightly bent and the spine curved inwards at the waist, which strains the abdominal muscles and throws the whole body out of alignment.

The myth that heels on shoes are essential is difficult to overcome, for the idea that the foot requires support has grown through the years. Many people really believe that heel-less shoes will cause fallen arches and other painful foot troubles. But if such support were necessary, surely nature, which has fashioned the physical body so exactly in other ways, would have put a further pad of bone or cartilage under the heel. The foot, wonderfully and intricately built, with tiny bones and muscles perfectly adjusted, must be made in this way to supply a definite need of the body; so would it not be wise to try to discover the right way to use the foot rather than to distort it for the sake of fashion and superstition?

Another way in which the modern shoe impedes the natural function of the foot is by unnatural pressure on the big toe-joint. The majority of shoes, particularly for women, are so built that the big toe, instead of forming a straight line from its tip to the instep, is pushed inwards at an angle, so that the joint is unable to function freely. Thus much of the flexibility needed in smooth and graceful walking is lost. When the intricate bone-structure of the foot is thrown out of alignment deformities and malformations gradually result; not only in the feet but in other parts of the body, owing to the whole being slightly out of balance.

It is difficult to find shoes which allow the freedom necessary for the foot's perfect development and functioning, although some of the modern styles for casual wear are fairly good. When choosing a shoe for constant wear, try to find one that is heel-less or only has the slightest heel, not more than half an inch. Whenever possible walk about with bare feet, or clad in soft slipperettes, or thick socks, making sure they are not too tight. It does not matter wearing shoes with small heels for special occasions, but for each day and all day it is important to give the body the correct balance and the foot the freedom and strengthening exercise which comes from walking without a heel.

Dr Scholl's Exercise Sandals (flat-heeled variety), which in the UK are obtainable from most branches of Boots and other multiple stores, are a splendid contribution to foot health. It may take a little time to grow accustomed to them, but it is worth following the directions exactly and only wearing them for a short time each day until the foot can manage them easily. After this they can be worn with comfort and pleasure practically all the time in the house and for casual outdoor occasions. The thick sole keeps the foot surprisingly warm, even in cold weather, probably because the constant movement which brings all the muscles into play keeps the circulation flowing freely. There are also good 'natural shoes' on the market now.

In choosing ordinary shoes, search for those with a practically straight line from the toe to the instep so that the joint of the big toe can move freely. If you trace the outline of your bare feet and then trace the outline of your shoe, you may well be surprised, on comparing the two drawings, to notice how much the big toe is pushed inwards. This means that it is impossible to give that final push from the ball of the foot which makes for speed and grace in walking.

It is difficult to walk correctly unless we do so either bare-footed or wearing a heel-less shoe or sandal which gives the necessary freedom at the big toe-joint. With the normal heeled shoe it is impossible to bring all the muscles and joints of the feet fully into play. It is therefore good often to practise walking with bare feet in order to gain some idea of the correct movements. Flexibility of the foot at the big toe-joint gives a smooth gliding movement that makes walking beautiful.

If you walk around the house in this way you will soon

notice that the knees are used differently. There is a stretch at the ankle and back of the heel which helps to straighten the knees in walking so that every stride is finished with the knee straight. The knee should be stretched at the beginning and end of every stride; as we step forward, with the front knee stretched, the heel only should lightly touch the ground, but as the weight rapidly passes over to the ball of the foot there should follow a slight springy push from the ball of the back foot and the toes, helped by the straightening of the knee. This impels the body smoothly forward and

6   Walking correctly. 'As we step forward, with the front knee stretched, the heel only should lightly touch the ground, but as the weight rapidly passes over to the ball of the foot there should follow a slight springy push from the ball of the back foot and the toes, helped by the straightening of the knee.'

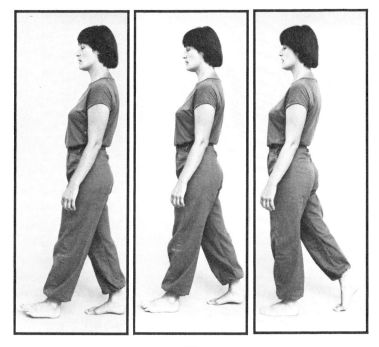

gives impetus for the next stride. The complete use of the foot gives almost a rolling movement from heel to toe which does away with any jerk in the walk. Walking thus with bare or lightly-clad feet, it will not be long before we are conscious that feet and knees are working more flexibly and naturally, bringing a sense of lightness and comfort which pervades the whole being – especially when we remember the 'Star-hook' which keeps the back of the neck freely stretched and the shoulders relaxed, down, down, down!

You will notice that the knees get much more exercise than they did before, when walking like this, as they are stretched with each stride; also stretched is the back of the heel, and one effect of this is to help loosen the pelvic muscles. We become increasingly aware of how each part of the body links with others so that misuse of one small part can throw the whole organism out of balance.

The habit of walking about with bare or stockinged feet and concentrating on the way the foot is working will bring increasing life and movement into the whole leg. The constant full stretching of the knees will bring into action some little-used muscles which will strengthen the joint, as will training ourselves to use the knees when bending to pick up something from the floor. How few people do this as they grow older! Watch the spontaneous activities of the healthy toddler; see how easily he bends the knees and squats down with the heels flat on the floor to play with a toy. With most people of mature years this seems almost impossible and we soon realise the need for some 'knees bend' exercises.

When training the knees to work properly, it is important not to try to force them in any way. The knee is a beautiful and complicated joint which can easily be damaged by strain or misuse; and so we need to work gently and carefully when trying to increase its flexibility. The gentle stretch of proper walking will start the loosening process and we can help the joints to become more flexible by swinging the foot from the knee whenever it is possible to do so. Sit on a table or a stool high enough to allow free movement, and just gently swing the foot backwards and forwards, thinking of the knee-joint. Remember always the importance of focusing the mind on that part of the body which you want to strengthen and bring into use. Incidentally, the extra stretch at the back of the heel which comes with practice of the sitting/standing exercise, with bare or stockinged feet, will also strengthen the knees and loosen the hip-joint (which is where the legs join the pelvis, and not in the middle of the trunk, remember).

In squatting exercises we are trying to form the habit of keeping the head, neck and spine quite straight while doing work that requires bending, or lifting something from the floor. This conscious control of the balance of head and neck will co-ordinate all the other bodily movements so that no undue strain is put on any particular joint or muscle. So, think your usual directions – 'Star-hook', shoulders relaxed, heart lifted and tail down under. Now with the feet comfortably apart stretch the toes and feel the sensation of the whole foot comfortably spread on the floor. Feel that you are absorbing the strength of mother earth.

Wriggle your toes and separate them. Take your mind to each individual toe and see if you can make it move independently of the others. Feel the arch of your instep and see if you can lift it a little. Control of the instep – the navicular bone – leads to controlled poise of the whole body – the navigation of the ship of both body and soul!

Now take your mind to the knees. Think of them loosely, flexibly, bending outwards, as you also bend at the pelvic joint. As usual, don't do the action, just think it: imagine your knees bending outwards easily, loosely, as you reach down to the floor to pick up some object. Hold the picture clearly, then think of the line of light from the shining Star above you, and relax . . . into the action. Don't worry if at first you feel stiff and awkward, try again. Go through the whole process – think – imagine – relax into the action, about five times. Do it regularly each day without fail, and before long you will find yourself almost instinctively bending the knees and squatting when you have some work to do on the floor or at a low shelf. When it becomes habitual to squat instead of curling over at the waist, there will be no more need for special practice of these small movements because you will be using them all the time, while the ankles, hips and knees will be growing steadily more flexible and comfortable. If you are overweight, the state of knees and feet will be greatly helped if you make a determined effort to get back to your ideal weight.

All the little movements previously described are gentle and perfectly safe to practise on your own provided that you follow the instructions and think them over carefully. Remember that it is tempting to rush spontaneously into action rather than to think and relax into each movement. But it is the thinking, the conscious effort to become aware of the small movements involved in an easy upright posture, in light graceful walking and deep energising breathing that will gradually bring the downward pull from the body-elemental into perfect balance with the upward pull of the body of light. These small movements, practised regularly with the floor or wall to guide and support the body, avoid the danger of the strains and tensions which can arise from the typical 'daily dozen'.

The exercises I have given form a simple and safe pre-liminary to the practice of hatha yoga, which can be wonder-fully beneficial. If you can manage to attend the class of a good yoga teacher trained in the Iyengar method, which takes the student through the classical asanas with great care for the overall balance of the muscular system, it will enable you gradually to develop for your physical body a state of flexibility and poise which you hardly believe possible at the moment. Yoga helps to discipline the soul into a state of peaceful surrender to the will of the spirit. A trained Iyengar teacher will also be able to assess your individual needs and guide you to practise those *asanas* which are most helpful to you individually.

Jenny Beeken, one of our White Eagle yoga teachers, has prepared a written course (see end of chapter) which sets out a simple and well-planned series of movements which will lead the student to a fuller understanding of each *asana* and its effect on body and soul. Whether or not you can attend classes this course is designed to remind you of the deeper purpose of each movement and help you to understand it more fully.

Physical practice and discipline in posture can also lead you into a deeper understanding of meditation, for in each exercise we are trying to 'practise the presence of God' within every cell of our own body. This is true *yoga*, the conscious union of the little self with the omniscient, omnipotent, omnipresent Power – Wisdom – Love – God – the I AM – the source of all healing. Once this realisation comes, nothing is impossible. But to reach it takes patient effort, entails 'keeping on keeping on'.

NOTE

If you are suffering from back pains or strains, or feel that you could benefit from professional help to bring your body into proper alignment, you may contact the Alexander Teaching Association, in your own country or at A.T.A. Centre, 188 Old Street, London EC1V 9BP (enclosing stamped addressed envelope), telephone 01-250 3038. The Association will give you the address of your nearest trained Alexander teacher and therapist. It is of course easier and quicker to progress under a good teacher who will assess your special needs, but if this is not possible, a combination of regular practice of the simple, safe movements I have described, together with spiritual healing, will benefit you greatly.

The White Eagle Yoga Course is obtainable from the publishers of this book. For price see latest list and order form, which will be sent on receipt of a stamped addressed envelope. Yoga classes and therapeutic sessions are held at several of the White Eagle Lodges. For details of these, as for the order form and list, please write to New Lands, Rake, Liss, Hampshire, GU33 7HY.

Those who are interested in the Alexander technique are recommended to any of F. M. Alexander's books, but particularly to *The Use of the Self* (Methuen, 1932); or, if preferred, to *Stand Straight without Strain: the original exercises of F. Matthias Alexander*, by Marie Beuzeville Byles (Fowler, 1978).

6

EATING FOR ENERGY

A S LONG AGO AS 1936 White Eagle was giving his students advice about healthy living. Some of this appears in his book *Spiritual Unfoldment I*. 'There are', he says, 'certain basic rules for physical well-being and spiritual training, which we will give you.

'One rule concerns what you should eat. You know that man possesses subtler bodies in addition to his physical body, and his food supplies nourishment to the different types of atom composing the physical and etheric bodies. If he eats the coarser foods he stimulates the coarser atoms. Whereas, if his tastes incline him to eat only sun-nourished foods such as fruit, ripened corn, nuts and vegetables he will feed and nourish the higher aspects of his being and thus assist his spiritual unfoldment. The eating of coarser foods will make his training harder and longer – that is all.

'From birth onwards to middle age and death the body is becoming congested with poisonous accumulations.

'The foodstuffs that civilisation has produced, when assimilated into your body, tend to produce this clogged condition. The water you drink also has this effect. Foods of the wrong type tend to thicken the bloodstream and cause in middle life and old age, much sluggishness. Your object, if you are on the spiritual path, is to purify the physical atoms; and if you want pure vehicles you must eat pure food.

'It is better not to eat flesh because so often animals are killed under conditions of fear, and the blood, the red meat, will transmit to you the fears and the coarse vibrations. You would be very horrified if it were suggested to you that you

68

should eat your brother at your side. You would think it a shocking thing, wouldn't you? There was a time when degenerate races did this but you regard it as a depraved taste. In a little while the eating of the flesh of any living creature will be considered depraved taste, quite apart from the cruelty inflicted. Cruelty is a very important subject and the one on the spiritual path steers clear of cruelty in *any* form.'

When White Eagle spoke these words, his immediate family and close friends were by no means vegetarians, but we were steadily working towards this way of life. White Eagle warned us to do this gradually so that the body would become accustomed to the new way of nourishment and enjoy it. If people feel deprived of foods they enjoy, they will only do without them for a time and then will be unable to resist the desire to return to the old way of eating. How many would-be slimmers have discovered this fact by bitter experience!

So towards the end of the 1930s we came to the stage of virtually cutting out red meat but still eating fish, poultry and bacon. Even these we would not eat regularly, but only if we felt a desire or need for them. We were beginning to realise how delicious well-cooked vegetarian food could be.

The times when we ate flesh foods became less and less frequent so that when the wartime rationing came into force we were able to register as full vegetarians.

When I had children, just after the war, as a conscientious mother I was naturally anxious that they should be adequately nourished, particularly with regard to vitamins A and D, so I re-introduced fish in the form of herrings into the diet, and occasionally chicken. However, neither of these foods proved popular. I found that the children were much happier eating cheese and nuts and when, at an early age, Rose told me that she could not possibly eat herring because she could not bear the look in its eyes, I gave up trying to feed them on fish.

In fact, Rose's subsequent career as a vegetarian cookery writer suggests that her remark at that tender age was the first indication of a soul-mission. I need not have worried. All Mrs Cooke's grandchildren and greatgrandchildren are more or less lifelong vegetarians, and their vitality and health seems to compare quite favourably with that of their meat-eating friends. It is obvious that Rose was in no way lacking essential vitamins and nutrients.

Anyone who has made a study of diet soon realises what a complicated and even thorny subject it is. There are so many theories, so many advocates of different régimes, that it is difficult to pick a wise and sensible route through them all. Our family have always enjoyed food itself and the creation of new recipes. In the course of this enjoyable occupation we tended to put on weight and would try the various systems for slimming that came into vogue and fitted in with our vegetarian principles. With tremendous efforts of self-discipline we would trim ourselves to a (nearly) desirable weight, and then as soon as our vigilance relaxed, steadily and inevitably the unwanted pounds crept back. It is difficult to enjoy food and to keep one's weight within bounds. I do not honestly think that people who put on weight are necessarily greedy. It is surely right to enjoy food, good food, and it seems ungrateful to the divine providence which provides it (and to the cooks who prepare it) not to eat it with relish.

It was during 1982, just before I began work on this book, that we were led to a system for our meals which seems for us personally – myself; John, my husband; and Ylana, my sister – to have solved our problem. We have come to recognise that it is not so much the amount of food we eat as the way the different foods are combined that seems to make us put on weight. We have discovered this through personal experience which has led us to appreciate the immense value to health of single-food meals. This seems a strange concept

70

to many people, but through experimenting with them we have had to acknowledge that the ordinary mixed meals of haphazardly combined foods which form the regular diet of most people can be extremely clogging to the system, and produce a sleepy, sluggish state of health (thus confirming White Eagle's words at the beginning of this chapter).

From babyhood we become accustomed to arranging our meals in a certain way, building upon food-habits which are traditional to our own social group. Thus we develop a pattern of consumption forced upon us by our environment, which the body adjusts to, whether or not these eating habits suit us as individuals. In time our natural likes and dislikes are added to or subtracted from the norm, but basically we tend to follow tradition. Unless we are diet enthusiasts or are forced through illness or discomfort to take stock of the situation, we think no more about it. We accept the pattern of eating (or over-eating!) as an ordinary part of life.

To some, food gives more pleasure than to others, and eating forms for them an important part both of relaxation and happy social life. They find delight in producing or partaking of tasty meals. Other people seem much more interested in various creative activities, their minds completely concentrating on some favourite project. Perhaps the second group contains the people who are most tempted by the ready-made foods in the supermarkets; and unless they are aware of the dangers they will find themselves gradually losing vitality or developing allergies as a result of the chemical additives in their food. It is interesting to notice that some people who are full of vitality and enthusiasm for life seem to exist on very little food. We jokingly say that a lettuce leaf and a caraway seed are all so-and-so eats for lunch. Yet in this absurd diet lies an element of value, for here is a combination of foods which are both pure and full of life-force, combining the nourishment of mother earth and the vital energy of sunlight.

71

For years followers of Nature Cure methods have advocated the value to health of fasting – but how many people in busy lives, especially people who enjoy food, will discipline themselves into planning even such a simple measure as setting aside one day a week on which they will eat nothing but fruit? This is nothing like as difficult as the severe fasts advocated in Nature Cure in which one is limited to water or lemon juice; but it is surprising how much cleaner the body feels after a 'fruit only' day. Try it. You can have as much as you like of any fruit but with one proviso: *eat only one kind of fruit at a time.* Think about it while you are eating it. Enjoy every bite, and as you eat, give thanks for the sunlight, the nourishment of mother earth and the labour of brother man which have produced the fruit. Some food reformers advocate keeping to the chosen fruit for a whole day so that it will have its full cleansing effect on the system. This is particularly true of grapes. When they are cheap and in season, to eat nothing but grapes (different varieties if you like), and plenty of them, is an excellent way of cleansing the system and of becoming more aware of the real needs of the body and how to release its different energies.

Many of us eat thoughtlessly, chattering with our companions or, if alone, while reading a book. In this state of unawareness it is all too easy to pack in too much food, haphazardly combined, and to finish the meal hardly aware of what we have eaten. That is, until some little digestive discomfort later reminds us that we have eaten not wisely but too well. Never mind, in goes a 'Rennie' and we soon forget about it. Eventually we see the sad results of this thoughtless eating building up in our own bodies and those of so many of our companions.

People vary so much in their dietary needs that we would hesitate to advocate a specialised form of diet which would suit everyone. Some people need much more protein than

72

others; some people, especially young people and those engaged in occupations involving much muscular effort, will need more bread and carbohydrate foods. Experience is leading me, however, more and more to the idea put forward by Dr William Howard Hay and many other researchers at the beginning of this century, that of eating foods in the combination in which they will be much more easily digested.

To discover the real needs of our own particular bodies, it is a good idea to start with a cleansing period of one or more fruit days each week, choosing ripe fruits in season, those which we really like. This will accustom us to the idea of the single-food meal. A whole week devoted to meals of fruit, one food. We do this in order to experience the effect of that particular food; to learn how much we really like it; learn for how long it gives satisfaction. It is surprising how much one can discover about one's own real likes and dislikes with the single food meal. A whole week devoted to meals of fruit, one fruit per meal but plenty of it, will cleanse the system and sensitise the taste buds to become more aware of the real goodness in food. All fruits should be ripe enough to be eaten without sugar or any sweetening. Wash them well and eat as much as possible of the whole fruit – skin, pips, within reason. In many fruits, every part has its value in cleansing and nourishing the body.

During this period of cleansing and retraining the taste-buds, drinks should if possible be restricted to pure water (bottled spring or filtered water rather than ordinary tap water), herbal teas or fruit juices. Artificial diet drinks loaded with sodium compounds should be avoided now and always. These drinks poison the body with artificial chemical compounds. If you have to do without your tea and coffee, you may think a long time before starting your diet experiments, so ease yourself in gently by taking your favourite drink in strict moderation. Weak China tea with lemon is virtually harmless as well as enjoyable. If you are fond of coffee, try to accustom yourself to the filter method (such as Melita), which gives you the good flavour without the harmful acids. You will probably find however that your fruit meals are so satisfying and give your mouth such a clean taste that before long you will want less tea and coffee and will find yourself enjoying plain water.

After a week of fruit meals you will probably be longing for a change yet feel unwilling to go straight back to the old pattern of eating. Now is the time gradually to introduce other pure foods: the simple, natural ones such as vegetables, salad in season, and whole-grain foods. Again you will find it an interesting experience to keep to your single-food meals except for the introduction of a little fat where required – for instance, butter (in moderation) with potatoes – which should always be cooked in their jackets and the skins eaten.

Potatoes on their own, as much and as many as you want, taken with a moderate amount of butter, make a satisfying and enjoyable meal and will not put an ounce on the scales. In fact you will be surprised at how quickly your weight will adjust itself with single-food meals. Try a meal consisting just of wholewheat bread (home-made if possible), again with a moderate amount of butter. Chew it well and enjoy every mouthful, thinking of the sunlit fields of golden corn, the angels of the air, the earth, the water and the sun who have brought these delicious foods into being.

It is surprising how much energy one can find after a good meal of fruit; most interesting, too, to discover which particular fruits are most personally satisfying. For instance I have found that a meal of apples (skins, pips, core, all eaten and nothing left but the stalk) is more sustaining than a meal of two or three bananas. Living in the country in the strawberry season is a real delight and I find that a whole day on strawberries (without sugar or cream) or cherries in season, can be delightful and extraordinarily energising. When peaches are at their cheapest, a meal of these (three to five according to size) provided what I can only describe as joyful energy for quite a long time. Soaked dried fruits can be included in the régime: prunes, figs, raisins or apricots (a meal of single fruits, not mixed) are satisfying and sustaining. With each fruit be sure to eat as much as you want and over as long a period as you want but have a two-hour break between the different fruits. If you are changing from a fruit to a different food-type allow about three hours between.

You will not, I believe, feel hungry, and if you can bring yourself to keep to these fruit meals for a whole week you will be surprised how clean and vigorous your body will feel, and how much more aware of the special quality and flavour of each of the fruits. If you take the fruits one at a time the vital forces in these natural products seem to be quickly released into the body and a cleansing, healing, nourishing process is set in motion. A régime such as this, provided that you carefully wash all fruits before eating them, will help to cleanse away the residue of chemical additives absorbed from processed foods.

Strangely enough, when foods are taken singly as described, the body seems able to concentrate the whole digestive process on the one particular food and to extract the maximum amount of nourishment and energy from it: more so than when it is mixed with several other foods. You have to experience this to believe it. Orthodox nutritionists will no doubt laugh at the idea. Until you have experienced the delight of feeling your body reacting to specific foods you will accept conventional ideas about nutrition, but when you start to experiment in this way with the single-food meal and later with blending foods that go harmoniously together, you will soon be convinced.

So – what really constitutes a healthy diet? We are often

asked if White Eagle insists that his followers all become vegetarians.

White Eagle does not dictate on this or any other matter but he does point out that (quite apart from the humanitarian aspect) a vegetarian diet wisely planned is not only the most health-giving but will also gradually refine the physical atoms so that they become more responsive to the subtler spiritual vibrations which we are longing to become aware of through spiritual unfoldment.

Jesus said, *Not that which goeth into the mouth defileth a man; but that which cometh out of the mouth, this defileth a man* (Matthew 15:11). In other words, what we eat does not matter so much as how we think and speak and act. Too much thought and concentration on the body and its requirements can be just as unfortunate in its results as too little. Nevertheless, certain principles hold good in any diet which forms a healthy way of life.

1. Only eat when hungry – when the body instinctively needs food. Most of us eat far too much as a matter of habit and routine. This is where the single food meals are so helpful in that they increase the awareness of the body's *real* needs.

2. Avoid eating if tired, lethargic, listless, in pain or in mental distress (unless your tiredness is due to lack of food!). In these circumstances the digestive juices are not working well and the food taken will stay too long in the stomach and intestines. Just rest, sip water, or practise quiet Star-breathing until hunger pangs return.

3. Eat slowly and chew each mouthful thoroughly, tasting and consciously absorbing the vitality – what in the East they call prana – in the food. This process will make one much more aware of the deadness of 'junk' foods and the chemically-processed products which line the supermarket shelves. Try to use only whole grains, fresh fruits and vegetables, free-range eggs and, where possible, untreated dairy

76

products. Cut down hard on salt and all sodium compounds (watch for the hidden salt in processed foods), and if you must have salt take sea salt or biochemic salt. Avoid refined sugar and white flour. If sweetening is really necessary use honey or raisins or dates. If you want further information, one of Rose's books is very helpful: Rose Elliot, *Your Very Good Health* (Fontana, 1981).

4. Observe the rules of proper food combination. The ideal rule is don't combine but eat one food per meal; but for many people this idea is strange and unappetising, though once you become accustomed to it, mixed meals seem much less attractive, and in practice are less satisfying. The next best thing to the one-food meal, and the one which is more practical in catering for the family, is the meal consisting only of foods that are compatible, and 'combine' well.

The theory of compatible food combining is not new. It was put forward in the early part of the nineteenth century by Sylvester Graham in his *Treatise on Bread and Bread-Making* (Boston, 1837), but the idea did not receive much recognition or popular attention until the early 1930s when Dr Hay formulated his system of compatible eating, the basic rule of which was, 'Don't eat proteins or acid fruits with starches (carbohydrates) at the same meal'. This became well-known as the Hay diet.

Since this time other researchers, especially in the USA, have advocated and developed this idea, until in 1982 it was brought to popular notice in the bestselling book, *The Beverly Hills Diet* by Judy Mazel (published by Sidgwick and Jackson). Judy, as I find I have to call her, does not write as a scientist or medical expert but as an enthusiast who discovered from her own experience that compatible eating, i.e. not mixing certain foods, could transform her constant ill-health to radiant vitality and reduce her gross overweight to true slimness. Naturally her friends were astonished by the results of her experiments and began to copy her ideas, which led to her writing her book.

We were made aware of the book's existence when last summer our daughter, Rose, always brought her own little pack of food when she came to visit us because she wanted to keep strictly to the régime laid down by Judy Mazel. We were intrigued by her persistence and by the unusual-looking dishes which she brought with her. We also noticed that she seemed to be glowing with health and energy. At the time my husband and I were both overweight. John was under the doctor for high blood-pressure, and I was beginning to accept constant rheumatic pains in the knees and shoulders as one of the inevitable trials of growing older.

Rose's strict régime lasted for five weeks but she was so impressed with it herself that she kindly gave us a copy of the book. I read and reread it carefully, my first reaction being, 'This is impossible! It's all very well for people living in California, but how do we in Britain obtain all these queer fruits, pineapples, mangoes, paw paws, kiwis, blueberries?'

Rose however assured us that she had little difficulty in obtaining these items from her local supermarket, Waitrose. So we started to look around, and soon discovered that if you looked for them these necessary items were readily available. As it was summer time and we live near 'pick-your-own' fruit farms, strawberries in quantity presented no problem and cherries were just coming on to the market.

One of the important rules is to make sure that you have plenty of the fruit stipulated for a particular day or period of a day so that you could eat as much as you could possibly want. You must never let yourself be hungry but always wait two hours before starting a different fruit.

As soon as we knew that we had at least a week's supply of the more unusual fruits we started. John has always loved fruit, and he was soon not only intrigued by the novelty of this way of dieting but thrilled by the way the superfluous pounds were dropping off. Both of us felt much less tired, were sleeping better and enjoying life. In summer time in England, specially when the weather is sunny, it is not difficult to live on fruit. This is how the first ten days of the diet were spent; ten days during which a thorough cleansing process seemed to be taking place. Perhaps the most difficult time was towards the end of the first week when we did feel a little depleted, especially on the days when we could have nothing but watermelon all day . . . not I may say the delicious honeydew melons, but plain old watermelon, the big green one with the rosy pink inside and hardly any flavour. I personally found this the most boring part of the diet, but important since its effect is to clear from the body all traces of the sodium and artificial chemicals which pollute so much and so many of our convenience foods.

The whole idea of the ten days on fruit is to awaken the vital forces in the body; to stimulate and feed them with the wonderful life-force to be found in the simple fruits.

After about ten days on what Judy Mazel calls 'mono meals' of fruit we were then led on to 'mono meals' of jacket potatoes, corn-on-the-cob, or four ounces at a time of almonds or cashewnuts. Each food, except for nuts, bread and butter which were quite generously rationed, could be eaten in unlimited quantity. After all that time on fruit, how we wallowed in a meal of unlimited potatoes baked in their jackets, with which we were allowed up to two tablespoons-ful of salt-free butter! We could have freshly ground pepper or any kind of fresh or dried herb for flavouring, but strictly no salt. This perhaps was one of the hardest rules at first for one's palate is so accustomed to salt that it takes quite a while before one begins really to taste and appreciate the delicate flavourings of the different vegetables. The other rule which I found really hard was no milk with tea or coffee. Nevertheless, even after the first few days, we were beginning to feel so much cleaner and livelier that we determined

79

to persist for the full five-week course. This régime is much easier if you are sharing it with a willing companion. I think it would be difficult to persevere through the various stages if one were cooking for a young family or had to stand up to the opposition of a partner.

During the second ten days of the diet we were gradually introduced to mixtures of food which Judy Mazel calls 'open meals', and it was at this point that we were made increasingly aware of three basic food-types which, according to this particular theory, should never be mixed. The three divisions are fruits; carbohydrates (this includes most vegetables: see below); and proteins, which Judy Mazel divides further into three sections: animal, fish and fowl; dairy proteins (cheese, milk, yoghurt); nuts and seeds. Some further notes:

Fats. Butter, cream and the various oils are compatible both with carbohydrates and proteins, but not, on this particular régime, with fruit.

Fruit. In this way of life fruit is always eaten at the beginning of the day, one fruit only and as much as you want. Once you have changed to another food-group you do not return to fruit until the next day. During the five-week course this rule became so ingrained that we have never wanted to break it. It is a way of life which we have found so completely harmonious that now practically always we start the day with a one-fruit meal, plenty of it, together with a cup of filter coffee and milk (we have now broken the milk rule without any ill-effects!). We try to have a different fruit every day, always fruits we enjoy, and we try to eat them with conscious and thankful appreciation, tasting and absorbing the life-force in every bite. When planning ahead we think in terms of a week at a time and try to have as much variety as possible. Thus when pineapples have been readily available and not too expensive we have each eaten a whole one for breakfast once or twice a week. On another day it will be apples or bananas or one of the dried fruits. After a thoroughly good meal of the chosen fruit we usually have a three- to five-hour break before going on to one of the other food groups. One day a week even now, however, we try to keep as an all-fruit day, or with fruit for the first two meals and a 'mono meal' of jacket potatoes in the evening because of the way it makes us feel – clean, light and radiantly full of energy.

Carbohydrates. This food-group includes all the different grain foods, i.e. foods made from wheat, rye, oats, maize, brown rice and any other (in our case whole) grains, as well as potatoes, root vegetables, green vegetables and all salads. It is this group which allows the greatest variety in 'open' meals and which can be developed into delicious mouth-watering menus. If one follows this plan of food combining, according to Judy Mazel's theory (which has certainly worked in our case), delicious carbohydrates like whole-wheat bread, corn-on-the-cob, jacket potatoes, artichokes and various pastas are not fattening even when eaten in quantity, alone or mixed with one or two other carbohydrates. It is only when mixed with protein that they seem to block up the system and cause overweight. In this class of foods we also have to consider the sugars, i.e. honey, sugar preserves, which are omitted entirely from the five-week régime, though fats, butter and oils can be eaten in moderation. If at all possible, we are advised to use untreated butter and cold-pressed oils because as soon as fats are heated the lecithin content which helps to digest them is destroyed. Untreated butter was unobtainable, but we still benefited from the régime.

Proteins. In this class the only foods that concern us as vegetarians are the dairy proteins (cheese, milk, yoghurt and eggs) and the nuts and seeds; but of course for non-vegetarians it includes meat, fish and fowl. The strictest rule of this particular régime, apart from not mixing protein with starch, is that once you have eaten protein in the course of the day, all other meals must be protein – so an egg for breakfast means protein all day. In effect this means that in meal-planning one tries to arrange for the protein meal to be in the evening, so that it can digest overnight, and be followed by a fruit breakfast. During the strict five-week period, cheese and milk were not allowed, so we found ourselves rather restricted on the few all-protein days, when we ate alternating meals of eggs, nuts and seeds. How we looked forward to the next day's pleasant variety of fruits and carbohydrates!

By the time we had come nearly to the end of our five-week régime, Ylana had become so intrigued with the change in our general health and well-being that she too decided to experiment with this new way of life. For this is what it is. It is not what we used to think of as a diet, although it starts with a few weeks of disciplined, thoughtful eating, planned to cleanse the body of the build-up of artificial chemicals, contained in so many processed foods, which rob them of their vital force. Occasionally during the five weeks the discipline seemed a little irksome, but we were beginning to develop a way of life which was so harmonious and so thoroughly enjoyable that we knew we could live with it permanently. During the last week of the diet some more or less ordinary, orthodox meals such as we had previously eaten were alternating with half or whole days on certain fruits. We soon realised that on the whole we enjoyed our delicious 'mono meals' of favourite foods such as jacket potatoes and butter far more than the variety of mixed foods in the orthodox open meal. There is now no doubt in our minds that certain food groups do digest much better on their own, no matter what nutrition experts may say. Since living on this régime neither of us has the slightest sign of indigestion. Elimination is greatly improved and we sleep better.

John's blood pressure is now normal and my aches and pains have vanished. Our friends all say, 'How well you are looking! I hear you are on some queer sort of diet. Do tell me about it. How I envy you your energy. Whatever are you doing?'

There is no doubt in my mind that this method of compatible eating awakens the life-force, the natural healing force inherent in the body, and brings a far greater enjoyment of food with an increasing appreciation of its life-giving properties. Strangely enough it has proved cheaper than conventional eating in spite of the tropical fruits.

Although the discipline is strict during the first five weeks, Judy also shows one how gradually to build a maintenance régime which includes your favourite foods. This is not a diet of 'never again apple pie and cream!' If you love apple pie and cream, you learn how to schedule it in, to enjoy it with abandon and then counteract any bad effects the next day by having one or more meals of a specific fruit. Judy gives a list of different fruits which she has found especially helpful for counteracting the ill effects of one's favourite foods.

The strange thing is that when you know that you can legitimately eat whatever you want, quite often you cease to want it! One's food tastes change and develop and the longer one is following this régime, based on natural, vital foods, the more one enjoys them. One loses the taste completely for the sugary, salty, highly-flavoured processed foods which form such a large part of the diet of our so-called civilisation.

The Beverly Hills Diet has been written with sincerity and enthusiasm for those who are troubled with overweight, and certainly for us it has worked with quite dramatic effect. It is, however, much stricter than the method of compatible eating taught by Dr Hay, who gave a really practical diet which can readily be adapted for family catering, and is equally health-giving.

In his book *A New Health Era* (Harrap, 1935) Dr Hay not only emphasised the importance of not mixing at one meal concentrated starches and acid fruits or concentrated starches and proteins, but also pointed out the need to maintain the correct acid/alkaline balance in the body.

One of the most helpful and enthusiastic exponents of his system is Mrs Doris Grant, who has written many books and articles on the subject, including the well-known and loved little book *Your Daily Bread* (Faber, 1944, but now alas out of print). In this she introduced the wonderfully easy way of making wholewheat bread without kneading, now famous as the 'Grant Loaf'. I am most grateful to Doris Grant and to the magazine *Here's Health* for allowing me to reprint the following extracts from a recent series of articles, entitled *Don't Mix Foods that Fight*, which throw further light on the question of acid/alkaline balance in the diet.

Readers may be interested to know that Doris Grant is a kindly supporter of White Eagle's work and in a recent letter writes:

'How strange to get a letter from you this morning as last night I was tidying my writing case and found myself re-reading a letter from your dear mother [Grace Cooke] . . . I felt so inspired after reading this letter and so encouraged. Your mother wrote "I am guided to tell you from White Eagle himself that your work is of great importance to humanity in preparing their physical bodies for the inflow of light and unfoldment which will come in the new Aquarian Age.

' "Although you may not know it yet, he knows you and says that you are one of the channels of the White Brotherhood behind the veil. They are using you to help humanity on to a purer and more healthful way of life . . . I have another impression, that we shall be very much linked with you in the future . . ." '

When I wrote to Doris with some questions about compatible foods, which she answered most patiently and fully, I had no idea that this correspondence had taken place. Here is the third of her articles:

'For optimum health and heightened resistance to disease the diet should, ideally, consist of alkaline-forming foods and acid-forming foods in the ratio, approximately, of four to one, which when metabolised will produce a corresponding ratio in the body. It is not difficult to distinguish between these two types of food. *Alkaline-forming foods* comprise all vegetables (including potatoes if cooked in their skins and the skins eaten); all saladings; all fresh fruits (except plums and cranberries); almonds; and milk. *Acid-forming foods* comprise: all animal proteins such as meat, fish, shell-fish, eggs, cheese, fowl; nuts (except almonds); all the starch foods such as bread and flour and other foods made from cereal starches.

'It should be emphasised that wholewheat and other whole grains are more acid-forming – and more rapidly converted into acid products – than all other foods, *including meat*; although good foods their intake should be kept low. Non-meat eaters, especially, should be careful not to overeat of starches in avoiding meat, otherwise their diet could be more acid-forming (and therefore less healthy) than one including animal proteins . . .

'As there is much confusion regarding the classification of acid fruits (grapefruit, oranges, lemons, berries, etc.) *as alkaline-forming* it should be pointed out, here, that the acids of these fruits leave the body within an hour or so of being eaten. They do so via the lungs (mainly), and the skin, urinary tract and bowel. The alkalies, when released from their combinations with the acids, provide a very valuable contribution to the body's alkaline reserve. Acid fruits can be acid-forming, however, and cause discomfort, when eaten at a meal containing high (concentrated) starches and/or sugars: in the first place they counteract the alkaline saliva in the mouth, and in the second place they neutralize the starch food's accompanying alkalies in the stomach. On the other hand, if acid fruits are combined at a meal alone with milk or yogurt, or at a meat and vegetable meal containing no sugars or cereal starches, they will not as a rule cause any discomfort.

'The best way to help achieve the ideal balance is to eat meat or other protein once a day only; to eat cereal starches once a day only (unless physically very active or very young); and to eat one meal every day consisting only of fruit, with milk – preferably as yogurt. Occasional days of *three* meatless [i.e. no-protein] and starchless meals are recommended . . .

'At this point it may be necessary to assure the reader that there is no question at all of sacrificing the delights of eating. Quite the reverse, menus planned compatibly and conscientiously, will actually increase the pleasures of eating as each menu is a complete contrast to the preceding one, providing stimulating variety. The diet as a whole, also, will inevitably contain a greater variety of foods of basically good quality than the diet, generally, of those on mixed meals. (While actually writing this section I received a letter from a recent convert to this régime in which she states ''I can truthfully say that we have never enjoyed our food so much as in the last few months and my husband still cannot get over his smoothly-working inside. Friends remark on how fit and well we both look''.)

'It will be found, also, that small, correctly combined meals are more satisfying and more nourishing, because better digested, than larger mixed meals, and create a marvellously comfortable and contented stomach, as the above correspondent's husband found in a very short time.

'It is not the amount of food that is eaten that counts but the amount that is properly digested, metabolized and absorbed by the body. In these days of incipient world food shortages and soaring prices, *more nourishment for less food* takes on a special significance.

'Most people in Westernized countries eat too much starch and protein. In the case of excess protein it has recently been established that this is not always eliminated by the kidneys as previously believed but can be stored up in the body cells, and is one of the main sources of so-called "over acidity" . . .

' "Disease", claimed William Howard Hay, "*is intrinsic to the body*", created by the body itself, through manufacture of more acid end products of digestion and metabolism than can be fully eliminated [. . . and he claimed] that if we understand better the self-created causes of many of our ills we can then do much more about keeping ourselves as well as we ought to be.

'An interesting analogy, here, is provided by the fact that the correct acid/alkali balance is also of importance *in the soil*. In the *Soil Association Journal* of December, 1973, Michael Blake stresses this importance and that the effect of an imbalance is not restricted to the soil, but is of "universal importance to all living organisms".

'That correctly combined meals are better digested than mixed ones was acknowledged as long ago as the early nineteenth century by Sylvester Graham in his now famous *Treatise on Bread and Breadmaking*.

'In this he states that although the alimentary organs of man and animals can be made to digest most vegetable and animal substances and a mixture of these at the same meal, they can without doubt manage one food at a time better than a mixed digestion. "Hence", he wrote, "it is a general law of nature, concerning the dietetic habits of man, that simplicity of food at each meal is essential to the highest well-being of the individual and the race."

'Sylvester Graham's statement that one kind of food at a time can be digested better than a mixed meal received strong support from Pavlov's research many decades later.

This showed that minced meat fed to a dog took 4 to 4½ hours to digest, but when this was mixed with starch there was a protracted delay; it took 8 hours before the food left the stomach.

'In *Thoughts on Feeding* Lionel J. Picton, MD, commenting on this delay as shown by Pavlov's findings, wrote: ''The somewhat startling conclusion flows from this that meals of a mixed character such as meat and bread, favour constipation, whereas meat and salad at one meal, and starchy foods such as bread – of course with butter – at a separate meal, have no such effect.''

'Today there are some seven million people in this country taking regular aperients at an annual cost of £16 million! Concerned physicians and surgeons have recently been warning that constipation can be – is – the forerunner of more serious symptoms and diseases. Recent research has shown that in the Western world the daily stool is less than half that of our rural Africans and Asians living on unrefined foods; that the consistency of the stool is hard and viscous and that the intestinal transit time (the time taken for the food to traverse the intestine) may be as long as *five days* (instead of 24 hours). Thus many people who think that they are not constipated may be very constipated indeed *in spite of having a daily stool*.

'Any delay in transit time can turn the normally friendly bacteria of the colon into unfriendly ones, even into virulent ones. These, in turn, create poisonous substances which are now linked with such disorders as urinary tract infections, arterial damage, and even with cancer of the colon. Carcinogens in food and in the environment are also linked with cancer of the colon, but as Dr Miles Robinson points out: ''Regardless of the cancer-causing agent the consensus is that the *longer* it takes the food to travel through the alimentary tract, the *more exposure* the colon will receive to the harmful agent.'' . . .

'A régime of whole foods correctly combined will ensure a beautiful and flawless complexion. It will also bring the overweight person gradually and safely down to normal weight without resorting to wearisome and sometimes dangerous slimming diets . . .

'Slimming diets merely deal with *the symptom* but do nothing to remove *the cause* – over consumption, in most cases, of devitalized refined food and haphazard, acid-forming combinations of these. The fact that this self-same diet brings underweight people *up* to normal, indicates that this régime is a *normalizing* one.

'The importance of a diet of unrefined, fibre-rich foods in preventing both over-consumption and constipation is now at long last being widely acknowledged, thanks to the widespread medical acclaim accorded to the concepts of Surgeon Captain T. L. Cleave. But these unrefined foods can be even more beneficial in preventing constipation if correctly mixed together . . .

'When meals are planned with regard to correct combinations the consumption of starches, and also of proteins, fats and sugars is *automatically reduced*. What is even more important, the consumption of the alkaline, base-forming foods, rich in the accessory food factors, is *automatically increased*, thereby contributing to the alkaline reserve and a well-balanced body chemistry.

'It has been argued that there is no need for us to bother about acids or alkalis as McCarrison's "healthy Hunzas" didn't know about these. (Sir Robert McCarrison is recognised throughout the world as the earliest and greatest medical pioneer in nutrition. See *Nutrition and Health* published by Faber and Faber Ltd). *There was no need for them to do so:* their nutrition and lifestyle were nearly perfect and vastly different to ours. By religious dogma they were restricted for food to the out-growth of the ground, with the exception of milk and cheese. Their diet consisted chiefly of fruits, nuts,

89

vegetables and wholegrain breads, thereby being high in alkaline-forming foods and low in acid-forming ones. And because meat was a rarity, their diet was practically exempt from acid-forming mixtures of meat and starch. The Hunzas also led a strenuous open-air life in the production of their foods which greatly contributed to an efficient digestive mechanism and to their general health . . .

'Few people who have conscientiously investigated the principles of correct food combinations and correctly applied them to their eating habits have failed to experience tangible benefits in a very short time. Those that have experienced these benefits enthusiastically adhere to this way of eating for the rest of their lives. In a recent press interview Sir John Mills was asked how he looked ''so astoundingly good at 70'' and why he had hardly put on a pound in 30 years. His reply: ''I've followed the same diet – the main rule is do not mix protein with starch – for 30 years.''

'During the first half of this century there have been a number of independent medical authors with sufficient insight and courage to challenge the prescribed conventions of our orthodox, haphazard eating habits, and to advocate the doctrine of correct food combinations: William Howard Hay; Frank McCoy; Herbert M. Shelton; N. Philip Norman; Lionel J. Picton; and Daniel C. Munro. These authors have all made valuable contributions to the interpretations of this doctrine, although some interpretations differ somewhat in detail and are not always practical for busy people.

'It is for this reason that William Howard Hay stands foremost among these authors for the present writer: his interpretations of the physiological principles involved are so eminently practical and ensure enjoyable eating for all the family which has no relation whatsoever to any kind of ''diet''. That eating should be truly enjoyable is of paramount importance, for – as a wise old physician has pointed out – "the preservation of health by a too strict regimen is a wearisome malady!" A certain measure of compromise in the diet, therefore, is infinitely preferable to insistence on carrying out rigid rules . . .

'Forty-five years' experience of the immense value to health *and* happiness of compatible eating has convinced me of a vital truth: that one can be as well as one wishes to be; health is man's normal state, he was designed, created, born to be healthy. This experience (and that of readers and friends) has also revealed beyond doubt that most illness is preventable being mainly caused by ignorance of basic food laws, or lack of discipline where eating and living habits are concerned.

'Lack of discipline is a largely contributing cause of many of the physical, mental and social evils of this present age. In *Man, the Unknown*, Dr Alexis Carrel, famous Nobel Prize winner, made a profound observation about the importance of discipline: "It is chiefly through intellectual and moral discipline and the rejection of the habits of the herd that we can reconstruct ourselves. It is a well-established fact that discipline gives great strength to man." In this same book Dr Carrel also made two other observations which are highly relevant to the present argument: "There is no doubt that consciousness is affected by the quantity and the quality of the food"; "The possession of natural health would enormously increase the happiness of man".

'In the light of these observations any self-discipline involved in adopting compatible eating habits takes on a new and wholly beneficial dimension for healthy, happy and successful living.'

Study of the following lists of compatible foods will make it clear that certain traditional food combinations are mostly to be avoided. Old favourites such as bread and cheese, biscuits and cheese, have to be replaced by apple and cheese or salad and cheese. Pastas are splendid mixed with tasty vegetables and herbs and as a starch meal can be valuable; but with cheese, no! Flesh-eaters can no longer enjoy the combinations of fish and chips, roast beef and Yorkshire pudding or sausage and mash, with a clear conscience. Vegetarians in some ways have an easier time following the Hay system because nuts and seeds, which supply much of their basic protein, combine with the concentrated starch, either of potatoes or whole grains. So vegetarians, if they wish, can enjoy potatoes with their nut roast, but only if it fits in with the rest of the day's planning.

FOODS THAT COMBINE WELL
(according to the research of Dr William Howard Hay)

LIST A

Proteins	Sub-acid fruits	Acid fruits
Eggs	Apples	Berries
Cheese (low salt)	Apricots	(strawberries,
Milk	Cherries	raspberries,
Yoghurt	Grapes	blackberries,
Nuts	Mangoes	etc.)
Seeds	Nectarines	Lemons
Sprouted	Peaches	Lime
legumes	Plums, etc.	Orange
and for non-		Pineapple
vegetarians:		Pomegranate
Meat, fish,		Prunes (Santa
poultry		Clara)

LIST B
Do not combine with foods in list A

Starches	Sweet fruits
Cereals, whole-grain	Dates
Bread, wholewheat	Figs

Flour, 100% or 81%
    wholewheat
Rice, brown unpolished
Oatmeal, steel-cut
    medium
Potatoes (cooked in skins
    and skins eaten)
Artichokes

Ripe bananas
Extra-sweet grapes
Raisins

Sugars (use very sparingly)
Honey
Barbados sugar
Molasses
Maple syrup (not
    synthetic)

LIST C
Harmonious with both lists A and B

All fats – butter, cream, vegetable oils, egg-yolks
Nuts and seeds
Raisins
All green vegetables and salad greens and herbs

Avocados
Aubergines
Carrots
Celery
Chicory
Courgettes
Cucumber
Fennel Root

Garlic
Green peas
Green beans
Marrow
Mushrooms
Onions
Peppers, green and red
Radishes

At first compatible food combining will need more careful thought and imagination on the part of the cook, but once the family are established in the new way of eating and members who have previously suffered from digestive discomfort discover how much more smoothly their insides are working, nobody will want to return to the old way of eating.

The first thing to do is to study the lists to get a clear idea of which foods are compatible, then analyse the family's favourite foods and the time of day when they like to eat these. Make a plan of a week's eating with these favourite foods written in for the appropriate days and times. Studying the list carefully, try to build a tasty meal round the favourite item by combining it with compatible foods. If the item is made of incompatible ingredients, there will probably be ways of adjusting the recipe to get a similar effect. Having done this, consider the rest of the meals for that day and try to ensure that there is a proper balance of acid/alkaline and raw/cooked food.

What is a proper balance? In *Your Daily Bread*, Doris Grant says, 'A balanced diet must not only contain all the necessary foods; it must contain them in the right proportion. This important fact is seldom recognised.

'To determine the correct proportion of different foods in your diet is quite simple. The body contains mineral salts, some acid, some alkaline. In a healthy body the proportion of alkaline to acid salts is in the ratio of 80% to 20%. If we would maintain this balance it is only reasonable to suppose that the foods we eat must yield, when burned up, alkaline and acid salts in the same proportion (i.e. four to one). The foods that yield alkaline-forming salts are all those which contain much water. The foods that yield acid-forming salts are all concentrated foods.'

Although this balancing of the acid–alkaline contents of the diet sounds complicated, in fact it works out quite simply. All you need do is plan one purely alkaline meal based on potatoes with salad or vegetables; one based on bread or grain products; and one based on a protein combined with compatible vegetables. For vegetarian cooks this resolves itself chiefly into being careful about cheese and eggs, making sure that they are used with compatible vegetables and also trying to ensure that only one meal each day includes grain foods. Children and active young adults, however, need and can assimilate more whole-grain foods than older people, who in many cases would be healthier and have more energy if they ate less. They should include in their diet many single-food meals from the alkaline range, which consists chiefly of all fruits and all the vegetable and salad items in list C. With imaginative menu-planning, it should be possible to lead the whole family into an understanding of proper food combining. This would be particularly helpful where there is a tendency either to overweight or digestive disturbance. Sensible food balancing and combining is *not* a diet – it is a way of life which will gradually normalise the weight naturally and pleasantly, without recourse to special diets. Let us now consider the different types of meal, to provide the proper alkaline/acid balance.

The Alkaline Meal

This should be a meal with no grain foods, sugar or proteins, for these are the chief acid-formers. Those who have experimented with the Beverly Hills Diet, or single-food meals as previously described, will probably find it easiest to make breakfast the wholly alkaline meal, choosing for this one different fruit each day, but plenty of it – enough thoroughly to satisfy the appetite. This, combined with a warm drink, makes a surprisingly sustaining meal.

Potatoes cooked in their skins make an excellent basis for a completely alkaline meal and people catering for school-children who want them to start a cold day with a hot meal could find these most useful, cooked in various ways. There are many interesting ways in which they can be combined with other vegetables or salads to make a most interesting and tasty meal, remembering always that any pudding or dessert should come from the fruits in list B, in this meal.

It is interesting that although most nuts are acid-forming, almonds are highly alkaline, as are dates and raisins. This fact is extremely useful to vegetarian meal-planners who are also watching the four to one balance, for these dried fruits with almonds can help to balance the acid of starch meals. Ripe bananas (they must be really speckled) are also highly alkaline, and can be used to balance the acidity of the grain meals, which is probably why bananas and dried fruits, together with fresh coconut (all alkaline) combine so agreeably with the rice used in curries, pilafs, etc.

For those needing to lose weight, Doris Grant recommends two or three days each week based mostly on the alkaline foods and cutting out the grain foods. Personal experience has taught us that the single-food meals in the alkaline category are extremely effective for weight loss. Since it is not easy to avoid eating the wrong foods, or wrong food combinations at times, it is a good idea to make a practice of at least one cleansing day (i.e., a wholly alkaline day) each week. For many people this is easier and more practical than a day's fast.

An understanding of proper food combining is particularly helpful to mothers whose children tend towards overweight, because it is a way of life which seems to normalise weight naturally, though it is important for these children to try hard to cultivate a liking for raisins, dates and the other sweet fruits instead of sweets, and also for home-made wholewheat cakes and biscuits rather than the usual white-flour products and junk foods in the supermarket.

With regard to butter and cream, Doris Grant writes in *Here's Health*, 'There is no need to worry about butter in moderation; a whole-food régime supplies the many nutrients necessary to its proper metabolism and conversion into energy.'

The Protein Meal

With non-vegetarians the distinction between protein foods (flesh, fish, fowl, cheese and eggs) and the starches is clearly defined, making menu-planning comparatively simple. During the course of the day one alkaline meal, one starch meal and one protein meal can easily be arranged. For vegetarians, however, there is a much more fuzzy edge between proteins and starches because, as Rose Elliot explains in her books *Beanfeast* (White Eagle Publishing Trust, 1975; alas out of print) and *The Bean Book* (Fontana, 1979) a combination of seeds, legumes or nuts with grain foods can provide the equivalent of what used to be known as first-class protein. It is for this reason that I recommend thinking first of the main meal of the day and planning the others round it. It is now recognised that our protein requirements are far less than was considered necessary at one time (White Eagle told us this forty years ago!) and when the meals are properly combined, the body seems able to extract more nourishment from the foods eaten so that even less is required. *One protein-based meal a day is quite sufficient* except for the young and those engaged in manual work.

Since nuts and seeds, two of the basic ingredients in the vegetarian diet, are compatible with both the A and B lists, the only protein items which we need to consider are cheese and eggs. Egg-yolks are compatible with starches – and indeed, for those who sometimes enjoy their scrambled, poached or boiled eggs with toast there is no reason why one should not 'bend the rules' sometimes and really enjoy these – but this should be done consciously and deliberately, and only on occasions – not all the time. (Remember, however, that nuts, with the exception of almonds and chestnuts, are acid-forming, so will affect the acid/alkaline balance.)

Cheese should be combined only with the salads and vegetables in list C, or the fruits in list A (specially apples). Cheese sauces for vegetables (as well as other sauces and gravies) can be quite tasty made with puréed vegetables instead of flour (recipe at the end of this chapter).

The Starch Meal

The basis of this is of course whole-grain cereals – whole-wheat bread, brown unpolished rice, pastry or cakes made from wholewheat flour and sweetened either with dried fruit or a little honey, also oatmeal, oatcakes, porridge, etc. If this meal is based on whole grains and plenty of fruit and vegetables are included in the diet there should be no need for extra fibre, but if it is felt to be necessary this meal can include a serving of bran in some form. The starch meal consists mainly of the above grain foods suitably combined with salads or vegetables and sweet fruits such as raisins and dates or ripe bananas. For hungry schoolchildren seeds and nuts can be included, almonds and dates being specially useful because of their highly alkaline nature. Delicious main meals are possible for those who are fond of pies or pastry. The imaginative cook can concoct tasty pies and flans combining the pastry with the vegetables in list C. Mushrooms are especially useful in this connection. Savoury pancakes are also popular. (If you want to be strict about proper food combining make them with egg-yolks only, and use the whites for making nut roasts or cutlets, for which in turn use wheatgerm instead of breadcrumbs, to bring them into the ordinary protein category and thus to be combined only with lists A and C items.)

Sandwiches of course come into this starch meal and the orthodox way of making them with a protein filling is hard on the digestion. Fillings should always be made from in-gredients in list C, which can be tasty and delicious, and sur-prisingly more satisfying than cheese or the flesh foods usually used. Again, if the children love egg sandwiches, bend the rules a bit, but do make full use of combinations of all the salad items together with ground or chopped nuts and raisins. (Remember the splendid alkaline balance of almonds with raisins or dates.)

Harmonious food combining is a way of life. Once the

rules become familiar, imaginative cooks can have fun thinking up the most delicious meals. This is not a régime of constant self-denial, but of rethinking the meals so that each one is based on family favourites with foods combined in such a way that more nourishment can be extracted with less tax on the digestion, and consequently more energy for enjoying life.

You may like to know that Doris Grant has written a new book with Jean Joice, *Compatible Eating for Health: a new look at the Hay System* (Thorsons, September 1984).

The following menus by Rose Elliot all involve combining compatible foods, and I am very grateful to Rose for contributing them specially for this book.

MENUS AND RECIPES

The plan of the following is that each day you will choose one meal from each category: alkaline-forming, starch and protein. It doesn't matter which order you take them in, though it is often easiest to make breakfast the alkaline-forming meal, leaving the starch and protein meals, which offer more scope for menu-planning, for later in the day. This means a breakfast based on fruit, natural yoghurt, almonds and raisins or dates, or baked potatoes in their skins. At lunchtime this could be followed by a starch meal of, for instance, salad sandwiches and a banana, and a protein meal such as cheesy stuffed aubergines with green vegetables followed by apricot fool for the evening. But this is a flexible way of eating which can be adapted according to your needs and fancies. You could, for instance, start the day with a starch meal of banana muesli and toast, followed by a protein lunch of salad with cheese, stuffed hard-boiled eggs or nuts, with fruit to follow, ending the day with an alkaline meal of jacket potatoes with salad or lightly-cooked vegetables followed by fruit. Make the meals fit in with your way of life and what your family like.

Once you understand the principles of the diet and know which foods are compatible, it is possible to adapt many recipes. Wheatgerm, which is classified as a protein, makes a good substitute for breadcrumbs in protein recipes, for coating rissoles, adding to stuffings or sprinkling on top of *au gratin* recipes, perhaps with some sesame seeds or chopped almonds (which are compatible with both protein and starch) mixed with it. Vegetable soups, made with vegetable stock, are also compatible with both protein and starch. If they are liquidised they do not need additional flour to thicken, although they can be enriched with egg yolk or cream for special occasions. An excellent sauce for serving with protein meals can be made from tomatoes. Soured cream and yoghurt also make delicious cold sauces, flavoured with fresh chopped herbs; while for special occasions traditional *sauce hollandaise* and *sauce béarnaise* can be served with protein dishes. Egg yolks can be used instead of whole eggs when making dishes for starch meals and honey can be used instead of sugar for sweetening puddings.

The following menu ideas and recipes show how these principles work in practice.

Recipes marked * will be found in my book *Your Very Good Health* (Fontana, 1981); those marked † are from my book *Gourmet Vegetarian Cooking* (Collins, 1982). For those marked § see below.

Alkaline-forming Meals

Breakfast
—Grated apple and natural yoghurt with raisins and chopped almonds.
—Banana yoghurt with sesame seeds and a little clear honey.

—Orange juice; mixed with fresh salad.
—Fruit compote* (use recipe in *Your Very Good Health*, with water or orange juice instead of the ginger wine).
—Baked apple with raisins.*
—Bircher potatoes* or jacket potatoes and butter.

Lunch or Supper

—New potatoes steamed in their skins with butter and chopped herbs, served with lightly-cooked vegetables; banana or grapes.
—Vegetable casseroie§; baked potatoes; yoghurt with clear honey and chopped almonds.
—Grated potato cakes§; cooked vegetables or salad such as cabbage, red pepper and carrot salad*; nuts and raisins.
—Jacket potatoes, chunky mixed salad bowl†, grapes.
—Carrot, apple and chervil soup†, mushroom, tomato and avocado salad bowl†, yoghurt and apricot fool (soaked dried apricots liquidised with a little honey and mixed with natural yoghurt and a little whipped cream).
—Carrot, apple, celery and raisin salad* with chopped nuts; fresh orange segments.

Starch Meals

Breakfast

—Banana muesli§; wholewheat bread or toast (the quick easy bread recipe in *Your Very Good Health* is fast and fool-proof).
—Chopped banana with dates and nuts; wholewheat bread or toast.
—Wholewheat scones* with butter.
—A muesli made of mixed whole flaked cereals, without apple but including nuts and raisins, mixed with cream, milk or natural yoghurt; wholewheat bread or toast.
—Natural yoghurt with raisins and nuts; wholewheat toast.

101

Lunches and Suppers

Packed Lunches. These can be based on wholewheat bread, rolls or pitta bread with fillings such as: grated carrot and raisins, bound with soured cream or home-made mayonnaise (without lemon juice, though malt or rice vinegar may be added); grated almonds mixed with chopped tomato; a spread made by liquidising sunflower seeds with a little oil and adding seasoning to taste; date purée; lettuce, tomato and spring onion; hard-boiled egg yolks mashed with cream or mayonnaise (as above); mashed banana and chopped almonds; yeast extract with sliced cucumber. A piece of wholewheat cake, such as the Dundee cake or date slices in *Your Very Good Health* can be included – or some nuts and raisins or dates and a ripe banana or sweet grapes.

Starters. Artichokes with butter; sliced avocado tossed in olive oil and chopped green herbs; tomato soup§; marinated mushrooms (from *Your Very Good Health* but omitting lemon juice); chilled cucumber and yoghurt soup (cucumber peeled and liquidised with natural yoghurt and a little cream and seasoning); sliced tomatoes with soured cream and chopped herbs on top; crudités served with a dip made from soured cream with chopped herbs stirred in; mushroom patties with yoghurt and spring onion sauce (from *Gourmet Vegetarian Cooking*, omitting cheese from pastry).

Main Courses. Vegetable lasagne§, buttered spinach.

—Vegetable biriani* with vegetable curry sauce* (leave out the hard-boiled egg garnish).

—Mushrooms on toast; side salad if liked.

—Herby pizza† (follow special pizza recipe in *Gourmet Vegetarian Cooking*, omitting cheese and topping with soured cream instead, or just adding extra herbs and olive oil; green salad.

—Vegetable casserole†, wholewheat garlic bread, or baked potatoes.

—Nutty brown rice with vegetables*, watercress.

—Onion flan§, lettuce, tomato and spring onion salad.

—Pasta with butter and chopped fresh green herbs; tomato salad.

—Mushroom pancakes§, green beans.

—Stuffed marrow baked with butter and thyme† (use just the egg yolk to bind and omit lemon juice and rind), roast potatoes, carrots.

—Nut roast – use any favourite recipe such as the white or brown nutmeat in *Simply Delicious* (White Eagle Publishing Trust, 1967), omitting the egg completely, or just using the yolks: it works well either way, but a little more water may be needed. Serve with vegetables, roast or steamed potatoes, and gravy.

—Chinese vegetables with almonds and rice*.

—Nut burgers served in a soft roll with salad – use the nut rissole recipe from *Simply Delicious*, using water instead of milk and leaving out the egg.

—'Devonshire Tea' or wholewheat scones* with honey and Devonshire cream.

—Special rice salad* with grated carrot and watercress.

Puddings. Egg custards, made with just the egg yolks; home-made vanilla ice cream†, using egg yolk version and single cream instead of milk, and honey instead of sugar; chestnut ice cream†, omitting brandy and using honey instead of sugar; banana muesli§, banana crumble§, grape brulée§, pancakes with maple syrup (use pancake recipe as given in mushroom pancake dish below); honey whip; baked bananas; dates filled with nuts.

Protein Meals

Breakfast

—Cheese and apple.

—Grapefruit, omelette.

—Stewed fruit and baked egg custard.

Lunches and Suppers

Packed Lunches. Hard-boiled eggs, devilled eggs (hard-boiled eggs halved, yolks removed and mixed with mayonnaise or cream and curry paste, then put back again) or cheese with salad; a piece of nutty flan with salad; cheese dip† (use cheddar cheese and red wine dip but use single cream instead of the wine) with crudités; cold nutmeat – use white or brown nut rissole mixture from *Gourmet Vegetarian Cooking*, using wheatgerm instead of the breadcrumbs; curried vegetable and nut pâté† with salad.

Starters. Vegetable soups without flour, such as the tomato soup§ given; avocado vinaigrette; grapefruit; Stilton pâté with pears†; stripey pâté†; curried vegetable and nut pâté with yoghurt sauce†; avocado dip* with crudités; avocado and mushroom salad*; cream cheese and herb dip with crudités*; marinated mushrooms*; pears with creamy topping*; creamy tomatoes with horseradish*; stuffed tomatoes*.

Main Courses. Vegetable casserole§, grated cheese; green salad with vinaigrette dressing.

—Nutty vegetable flan, green beans and buttered carrots.

—Nut burgers with fresh pineapple rings – use nut rissole mixture from *Gourmet Vegetarian Cooking* with wheatgerm instead of breadcrumbs; chunky side-salad of lettuce heart, celery and cucumber in vinaigrette dressing.

—Aubergines with mushroom and parsley stuffing*, sprouts, purée of carrots.

—Green peppers halved, steamed, then filled with fried onion, mushrooms and grated cheese and baked until golden brown; served with fresh vegetables and tomato sauce*.

—Curried eggs – use vegetable curry sauce recipe from *Your Very Good Health* but omit potatoes and add 6 halved hard-boiled eggs just before serving; serve with steamed and buttered cabbage.

—Nut rissoles in tomato sauce – from *Gourmet Vegetarian*

Cooking, using wheatgerm instead of breadcrumbs; green beans.

—Omelette with spinach.

—Fruit salad with curd cheese dressing*.

—Nutmeat with apple sauce – use the nutmeat given for the walnut pâté *en croute* in *Gourmet Vegetarian Cooking*, omitting chestnut purée; bake in a loaf tin and serve with a thin apple sauce and buttered sprouts, carrots and French beans.

—Colourful mixed salad with grated cheese; lettuce, cucumber, grated carrot, sliced tomato, spring onion, grated or cooked beetroot, sliced apple, raisins, celery, as available.

—Spinach Roulade† – use recipe from *Gourmet Vegetarian Cooking* but just omit the small quantity of cornflour or arrowroot from sauce and use double cream instead of single; serve with fresh vegetables.

—Ratatouille†, with grated cheese and buttered cabbage.

Puddings. Baked apples with raisins*; apricot fool*; summer fruit salad*; tropical fruit salad, omitting banana*; orange and pineapple compôte*; egg custard, honey whip, vanilla ice cream as for starch meals, see above; pears baked in honey; stuffed pineapple halves†; apple snow*; fruit fools made by stewing fruit with honey, liquidising then adding whipped cream; cheesecake made on a base of chopped nuts and ground almonds instead of pastry; fruit sorbets and water ices made with honey instead of sugar.

Recipes

FRESH TOMATO SOUP
(serves 4)

1 onion, peeled and chopped	50 g (2 oz) butter
900 g (2 lb) tomatoes, skinned and chopped	
700 ml (1¼ pints) water	
dash of sugar	salt and pepper

a little cream and chopped fresh basil or chives to serve

Soften the onion in the butter in a large saucepan over a gentle heat. Add the tomatoes and cook for a further 3–4 minutes, then stir in the water. Bring to the boil, then lower heat and simmer gently for 15–20 minutes, until the tomatoes are tender. Liquidise, then season with sugar, salt and pepper. Serve in individual bowls with a spoonful of cream and a little chopped basil or chives on top of each.

GRATED POTATO CAKES
(serves 4)
450 g (1 lb) potatoes, scrubbed
2 tablespoons wholewheat flour
2 egg yolks
salt and pepper
oil for shallow frying
Grate the potatoes fairly coarsely. Add the flour, egg yolks and seasoning to taste. Fry rounded tablespoons of the mixture in hot shallow oil; drain on kitchen paper. Serve immediately.

ONION FLAN
(serves 4–6)
150 g (5 oz) plain wholewheat flour
75 g (2½ oz) butter
1–2 tablespoons water
for filling:
350 g (12 oz) onions, peeled and sliced
25 g (1 oz) butter
150 ml (¼ pint) soured cream
2 egg yolks
salt, pepper and grated nutmeg
Make the pastry: sift the flour into a bowl, adding also the residue of bran from the sieve. Rub in the butter until mixture resembles fine breadcrumbs, then add water to make a dough. Roll out and line a 20-cm (8-in) flan tin.

Prick base; bake for 15–20 minutes until crisp. Reduce oven setting to 180°C (350°F), gas mark 4. While flan case is cooking, make filling. Fry the onion gently in the butter until soft but not browned – about 10 minutes. Remove from heat and add cream, egg yolks and seasoning. Pour into flan case and return to oven and bake for 30 minutes.

NUTTY FLAN
(serves 4)
50 g (2 oz) wheatgerm
175 g (6 oz) almonds or other nuts, ground
1 onion, grated
2 tablespoons oil
salt and pepper
for filling:
2 onions, peeled and chopped
25 g (1 oz) butter
225 g (8 oz) button mushrooms, washed and sliced
2 tablespoons cream
salt and pepper
50 g (2 oz) grated cheese

Set oven to 200°C (400°F), gas mark 6. Put wheatgerm, ground nuts, onion and oil into a bowl with a little seasoning and mix together. Press mixture into a well-greased 20-cm (8-in) flan tin, to cover base and come up the sides, like a pastry flan case. Press down well, then bake for about 30 minutes, until crisp and lightly browned. Meanwhile fry the onions in the butter for 7 minutes, then add the mushrooms and fry for a further 2–3 minutes, until just tender. Remove from heat, add cream and seasoning. Pour into nutty flan case, sprinkle with grated cheese. Return flan to oven for 10–15 minutes, until cheese has melted and lightly browned.

Another good filling for this flan is a home-made ratatouille mixture, again with a topping of grated cheese or with soured cream and egg yolks poured over, as for the lasagne recipe below. This needs to be cooked for about 30 minutes, until set.

VEGETABLE LASAGNE
(serves 4)
450 g (1 lb) aubergines
salt
1 onion, peeled and chopped
3 tablespoons oil
pepper
125 g (4 oz) dry lasagne
450 g (1 lb) tomatoes, skinned and sliced
300 ml (½ pint) soured cream
2 egg yolks
Wash aubergines and remove stalks. Cut aubergines into 6 mm (¼ in) dice, sprinkle with salt, put into a colander, and leave for 30 minutes, to draw out bitter juices. Then rinse aubergines, squeeze dry. Fry the onion in the oil for 10 minutes, add aubergine and cook gently, covered, for about 20 minutes, until aubergine is tender. Season with salt and pepper. While aubergine is cooking, prepare lasagne. Bring a large saucepanful of boiling water to the boil, add lasagne and boil for about 10 minutes, until tender. Drain. Set oven to 200°C (400°F), gas mark 6. Put a layer of lasagne into the base of a shallow greased ovenproof dish. Arrange half the aubergine on top, then half the tomato. Cover with more lasagne and repeat layers, ending with a final layer of lasagne. Mix cream with egg yolks, and pour over the top of the lasagne. Bake for 40–45 minutes.

VEGETABLE CASSEROLE
(serves 2–3)
2 onions, sliced
3 tablespoons oil

1 garlic clove, crushed
1 green pepper, de-seeded and chopped
225 g (8 oz) carrots, scraped and sliced
450 g (1 lb) courgettes, washed and sliced
2 sticks celery, sliced
225 g (8 oz) tomatoes, skinned and chopped
salt and pepper
chopped parsley

Fry the onions in the oil for 3–4 minutes, then add all the remaining vegetables. Cook very gently, covered, for 20–25 minutes, until all the vegetables are tender. Stir from time to time to prevent sticking. Season with salt and pepper. Sprinkle with chopped parsley before serving.

MUSHROOM PANCAKES

(serves 4)
125 g (4 oz) wholewheat flour
pinch of salt
1 tablespoon oil
2 large egg yolks
250 ml (9 fl oz) water
for the filling and topping:
450 g (1 lb) button mushrooms
25 g (1 oz) butter
300 ml (½ pint) soured cream
2 egg yolks
pepper

To make pancake batter put flour, salt, oil and egg yolks into a bowl. Gradually add water and beat to make a thin smooth batter, thinner than single cream. Heat a little oil in a frying pan, pour off excess. Add a couple of tablespoons of batter mixture, tip pan so mixture coats base thinly. When set, flip pancake over with a palette knife and cook other side. Remove pancake on to a plate; repeat process until all the mixture has been used and you have 8–10 thin pancakes. Set oven to 200°C (400°F), gas mark 6. Make filling; wash and chop mushrooms, then fry them in the butter for 5–7 minutes, until tender. Drain off any excess liquid: save this for stock. Season mushrooms, then divide between the pancakes and roll them up. Place pancake rolls side by side in a shallow greased ovenproof dish. Mix cream and egg yolks, pour over pancakes. Bake for 25–30 minutes.

GRAPE BRÛLÉE
(serves 6)
450–700 g (1–1½ lb) very sweet grapes
1 tablespoon runny honey, optional
275 ml (½ pint) double cream
demerara sugar

Wash grapes, halve and remove stones. Put them into a shallow dish that's suitable for putting under the grill. Drizzle the honey over the grapes if you think extra sweetness is required. Whip the cream until it stands in soft peaks, then spoon on top of the grapes, smoothing it evenly over them. Cover with a light but even layer of demerara sugar. Heat the grill to moderate; put the grape mixture under the grill until the sugar melts. Remove from the heat; cool, then chill for several hours before serving.

HONEY WHIP
(serves 4–6)
3 egg yolks
2 tablespoons runny honey
275 ml (½ pint) whipping cream

Put the egg yolks into a medium-sized bowl set over a saucepan of boiling water (see that the base of the bowl does not touch the water). Add the honey and whisk until mixture is pale, light and fluffy. Alternatively, you can use a table electric mixer, in which case you do not need the boiling water. Allow mixture to cool slightly while you whip the cream until it stands in soft peaks. Fold cream into egg yolk mixture. Divide between 4 or 6 small glasses and chill for 1 hour before serving. Serve with home-made shortbread biscuits.

BANANA CRUMBLE (from *Rose Elliot's Book of Fruit*, Fontana, 1983)
(serves 4)
4 bananas
125 g (4 oz) wholewheat flour
50 g (2 oz) ground almonds
25 g (1 oz) butter
50 g (2 oz) soft brown sugar
25 g (1 oz) flaked almonds
Set the oven to 190°C (375°F), gas mark 5. Peel and slice the bananas and arrange them in a lightly-greased, shallow ovenproof dish. Put the flour and ground almonds into a bowl and mix in the butter, using a fork: the mixture should look like breadcrumbs. Add the sugar and flaked almonds and scatter over the top of the bananas. Bake in the oven for about 20 minutes. Serve with cream or natural yoghurt.

BANANA MUESLI
(serves 1)
2 rounded tablespoons rolled oats
3 tablespoons cream
1–2 teaspoons runny honey
1 banana
a few chopped almonds
Put the oats, cream and honey into a bowl and mix to a smooth creamy consistency. Peel and slice the banana, add to the oat mixture. Spoon into a bowl, sprinkle with a few chopped almonds and serve at once.

7

LEARN TO UNDERSTAND YOUR OWN RHYTHM AND OVERCOME FATIGUE

HARMONIOUS LIVING, the key to good health, is largely a matter of adjustment between man and his environment. No two people have exactly similar bodies and temperaments nor the same needs. A course of action which suits one may well be disastrous for another. The simple rules of health so far described can profitably be followed by all, but they need to be adapted to individual requirements. Everyone has some sensitive and vulnerable spot – digestion, heart, nervous system, back, bloodstream, throat, ears, eyes, where over-strain will first manifest as pain or faulty functioning. This is nature's warning system, for as soon as failure occurs in the weak spot, we know that in some way we are breaking the health laws of our own being and must take steps to deal with the situation.

Many will say that because of the conditions in which they are placed, they have to ignore stress symptoms and plough on. This is a short-sighted policy, for quite often a little thought will reveal sensible ways of harmonious adjustment to personal strains and stresses. Instead of people allowing themselves to be swept along by a tide of small circum-stances which they think are beyond their control, they could, by only a little self-discipline, achieve greater harmony and adjustment, resulting in better health and more energy.

The first essential for everyone is to recognise their own normal quota of energy and to understand its rhythm. We all have a peak energy period during the twenty-four hours.

Our vital forces ebb and flow rather like the tides, and one of the important rules for adjustment is to recognise the periods of the day when we can tackle difficult tasks with equanimity, and the periods when, with energies at a low ebb, we need more restful occupations, those which do not require so much willpower and grip. Although many people are forced by circumstances to follow a fairly rigid routine, within this framework, with a little careful thought and analysis of the situation, it may be possible to organise things so that the jobs requiring the greatest amount of effort and skill are tackled when the tide of energy is rising or at its peak.

Fatigue is the greatest enemy of health and happiness. Not the tiredness which is the result of a good day's work well done, bringing a glow of accomplishment followed by deep, refreshing sleep: this is part of a healthy rhythm of life. But there is a fatigue which is cumulative. It is the result of many small strains, physical, mental and emotional, which build up over the months and years, causing a deep soul-weariness which robs life of its joy and colour. This type of fatigue comes both to the young and the old, though as we grow older we may have less resilience and so feel more hopeless about it. Deep-seated fatigue needs more than a good night's sleep, or even a month's holiday, to put it right, for it arises from soul-stress and, like sickness or bereavement, is one of the factors of life which force the soul to turn to the eternal Source for help and alleviation.

A potent cause of fatigue and lassitude is resentment, which is all the more insidious because often we are unaware that it lurks in the subconscious self. We think we are living tranquilly and tend to hide, even from ourselves, the sore spot which is blocking the life-force. It could be a little jealousy or discontent. It could be a hurt due to some quick-tempered remark of a partner or friend spoken in the heat of the moment. It could be sheer weariness with the pressures of life. One such example is that of the mother of a baby or toddler below school age who keeps her active day and night. Giving everything to the family, she may feel so weary that she has no energy or enthusiasm for a normal, happy sex-life with her husband. This can then lead both of them to build up emotional resentments, as they fail to understand each other's needs, and can make what should be a happy period of the life a time of petty argument and emotional outbursts due to frustration. At this period of life the support of a closely-knit family is much needed, but the material demands of modern life often make this impossible.

Kindly grannies or aunts (even adopted ones) are invaluable at this time, giving regular help with the children to allow mum a chance to get sufficiently rested and refreshed to have some emotional energy left to give her husband. A happy relationship in marriage is a source of comfort and strength to both partners, the warmth and tenderness radiating out into the family and beyond.

A similar situation may afflict young husbands, worn out with the competitive struggles of business life. The constant strains and pressures of each day leave them with no energy, so that they suffer a temporary lack of sex drive, which may amount to impotence. This condition calls for tender understanding and patience from the wife, who needs at such times to be able to give the calm loving reassurance of a warm, sensitive mother, rather than the emotional demands of a wife. Such a mature, selfless attitude can greatly strengthen and deepen the bond of affection between them and result in a truly happy outcome.

Many are the sources of deep emotional strain and fatigue within the family at different periods of life. Conflict between strong characters – the emotional demands of someone deeply loved – may be the cause of an inner conflict which is robbing life of its zest. If fatigue is such that even a good night's sleep still leaves us weary and lifeless it is worth while trying quietly to analyse the situation to see if we can pinpoint the cause. Honest self-analysis should bring to light the sharp little thorn around which the wound is festering; but we may need the help of a wise, loving friend or counsellor. Once the real difficulty is recognised and accepted, it becomes easier to cope with. A sense of humour helps to put the whole matter into perspective and quite often a little re-arrangement of the life or a heart-to-heart talk with the person concerned will relieve the pressure. Often it is the small, disorganised parts of our life that allow pressures to build up. The big, inevitable difficulties and frustrations which come at times into everybody's life can often be borne with more patience and equanimity than the small inharmonies in daily routine.

Another potent source of inner tension and strain is the lack of a satisfactory sex relationship: a broken marriage; a partnership which does not materialise; love which is unrequited. Although sex is the foundation of a good marriage and one of the cornerstones of a normal, happy life, it is far from being the most important or the only way to find fulfilment. Happiness in love and marriage is largely a matter of karma and also of the particular mission that a soul has chosen in this day of life. Some souls return to earth with special work to do, some special gift to give to a cause or to one of the arts; which means that all their strength and devotion needs to be focused in a certain direction, leaving them no opportunity, and possibly no desire for normal family responsibilities. For as soon as a couple come together in partnership, especially a partnership which produces a family, they take on important responsibilities which will demand their energy and attention for many years. Any gifted soul whose life is dedicated to one of the arts or to some specialised form of service, needs either to be free or to have a partner selfless enough either to understand their partner completely or to dedicate themselves to the needs of the artist or the mission.

If your karma seems not to be allowing you to find the perfect love, or the emotional satisfaction you think is your due (and in this your lot will be identical with millions of others) then for the present you need to widen your interests and to find ways of channelling your energies in some form of service, which will (in time or in a different way) earn for you the longed-for reward. It seems to be a law of life that happiness on any plane of being has to be earned. It comes as a by-product of dedicated service and accepting tranquilly and cheerfully the responsibilities of one's karma.

If the normal, happy expression of sex seems to be denied and the longed-for partner does not materialise, and you can find some kind of activity that you really enjoy, accept its disciplines and challenges so that you become increasingly absorbed and dedicated. If you love children or feel a special sympathy with some social problem, make opportunities to work and serve in this direction. Let your heart lead you and then become really involved. Don't play at it but really give yourself, and you may well find that you have a special work to do which will open up a most interesting path of service and fulfilment, and even draw you to the companion you are longing for.

Try also to be honest with yourself about your emotional responses, and avoid those things which overstimulate the desire-nature. Try to accept that there is a wise purpose behind your present frustration, and take a long, broad view of the situation. The physical body may be clamouring for satisfaction; the desire-nature may be filled with resentment that you cannot have your own way at present. But you – the real YOU – the shining, eternal spirit – are not your body, or your desire-nature. You – the real YOU – *know* that life is bigger, broader and infinitely more beautiful than the wilful, little body-self realises. You – the real YOU – can with prayer and aspiration learn to draw upon that deep, inner centre of strength and peace which will help you to channel the sex energy into some form of service or creative work. Sometimes there is a very deep vocation involved. Remember the wonderful inspiration of Gandhi, the teacher and saint, who with the loving co-operation of his wife, deliberately became celibate, channelling all his sex energy, his life-force, to give him the soul-strength to lead India to freedom. A mighty task he set himself, but it is this kind of dedicated service that the wise direction of the life-force can give the power and wisdom to sustain.

If you find yourself at times being overwhelmed with physical desire and longing, you may be helped by chapter eight of my book *Why on Earth* (White Eagle Publishing Trust, 1979). 'In Yoga the control of the sex fire is well understood and there are certain exercises, particularly a simple breathing exercise, which can be very helpful to those with lack of an adequate outlet for the sex energies.' The exercise I give is from Indra Devi's book, *Forever Young, Forever Healthy* (A. Thomas, 1955). You begin with a routine of relaxation and deep-breathing as described above in chapters two and three of this book. Now, 'Having taken five or six . . . breaths, close your eyes and try to visualise a great vital force operating within and outside of you. Concentrate your mind on it, keeping away any thoughts connected with sex. Now resume again the deep rhythmic breathing and do the following: each time you inhale, imagine you draw the sex energy upwards from its center, like a pump drawing up water from a well, and each time you exhale, direct it to the solar plexus [which is the energy battery of the body, where life-force is accumulated]. Or, if you prefer, direct it to the brain to be stored there. Keep on doing this exercise for a few minutes without interrupting the rhythm of your breath. If you haven't done any deep breathing before, stop this exercise as soon as you feel dizzy and resume it only after three or four hours. Simple as it may seem, its practice is very effective. It is essential, of course, to do the deep breathing correctly and to be able to will strongly that the sex energy should rise upward before being directed to the solar plexus . . . The combined practices of this exercise, the Yoga postures and breathings will not fail to produce soon the desired results, especially if you watch your diet and cut out all drinks and foods which act as stimulants.' Also firmly avoid conditions and situations which make emotional control more difficult for you.

Although everyone at some time has to face major problems of sorrow and suffering, often it is the constant niggling cares that are the source of strain and fatigue. Fear and worry dissipate energy and the worriers forget that by their negative thought they create vibrations liable to attract the very event which they fear. Sometimes the fears are vague and nameless, even trivial and petty, yet they become bogies which drain the vitality and rob the soul of joy. The only real answer to fear is the cultivation of a sure faith in the love and goodness of God. This to many people may seem too difficult, especially when they are confronted by the headlines in the daily press.

The finest way to counteract this battering of the outer world and the cumulative fear-thoughts which hang like clouds over humanity, is for the individual to make time at regular intervals during the day to withdraw from the outer consciousness to the still centre within the heart. Practise the Star-breathing and focus the mind on the eternal and infinite power of God: on the mighty rhythms of the universe and on the divine law which holds all things in harmony, which restores balance and brings order out of chaos.

When any injury occurs to the physical body the healing forces inherent in nature flow to the spot to rebuild and repair broken tissues. In exactly the same way, when the soul faces major trouble and catastrophe, it automatically draws to itself invisible forces, angelic powers which give the strength and courage to carry on. History affords many examples of the indomitable spirit of Christ which lies deep in the heart of every human being. No matter what disaster, sorrow or sacrifice has to be faced, there is a fund of universal strength and healing upon which man can draw. Major tragedy, however catastrophic it may seem, always heralds the beginning, the foundation of a new and fuller understanding, a life of richer happiness.

If constant fear and worry are robbing life of joy and interest for you, then daily, hourly, build into the sub-conscious mind this faith and confidence in the ultimate goodness, the wisdom, the power of God. Every soul has at some time to fight and win their own battle of the shadows. Star-breathing, with frequent repetition of some uplifting words such as those of the Twenty-third Psalm, will be found most helpful, especially just before sleep and on waking. A feeling of thankfulness for all the ordinary things of life should be cultivated. Few people train themselves consciously to appreciate all God's gifts which bring joy to living. In fact these blessings are only recognised when some unfortunate circumstance removes them. Let us then daily give thanks for air and sunlight, for rain and all the beauty of the countryside and garden, for shelter, for the ability to enjoy good companionship, music, beauty. This spirit of thankfulness comes more easily on some days than on others, but when the shadows of fear, depression and self-pity gather, again it is often helpful to repeat some uplifting words of thanks and praise, and to keep on repeating them like a mantram, *'Praise the Lord, O my soul; and all that is within me, praise his holy name'.* This positive effort of thankfulness opens a pathway of light through the dense fog of self-pity down which the angels of healing can come to minister to the soul.

Another cause of cumulative fatigue is when, through excessive desire to be useful or to make the most of life, we try to pack too much into the daily routine. This indicates the need to control over-enthusiasm or a greed for living; to become more attuned to the great rhythms of eternity, which bring a sense of peace in the realisation that all things can be accomplished in God's good time. We defeat our own ends by working at such pressure that we allow no time for the springs of energy in our being to replenish us. To live harmoniously, we must accept and live within our own energy-rhythms, allowing due time for restoration and refreshment. When this law is broken, nature eventually steps in, forcing a longer break and disrupting our schedule far more than if we had worked at a gentler pace.

It is a good idea to form the habit of relaxing frequently all the time we are about our work. When concentrating hard on the task in hand, we almost automatically tense brow, jaw, shoulders and possibly hands and wrists. It is helpful to plan some little signal such as the clock striking which will remind us to relax for a few moments, to recognise the mounting physical tensions and concentrate on releasing these by taking a few moments off for Star-breathing. Think first of straightening up the posture ('Star-hook'; neck freely stretched; shoulders relaxed down; heart open to the Sun). Slow down the breathing and for a few moments either think of the Star and radiate the Light or just imagine some place or object of beauty which you find restoring. This may be the music of the seashore, of a singing stream or waterfall, of wind in the trees; it may be the form and fragrance of a flower or the thought of the loving affection of child or animal. Cultivate a 'homing' thought which will give you a few moments' respite in your task.

If you are tense physically, and conditions permit you to do so, raise your arms above your head and grasp each elbow with the other hand. Stretch up, then loosely relax forward and down. Let the weight of your head and arms pull down to give your spine a good stretch and relax in this position for as long as you can. You will find that on

120

straightening up again you return to your task refreshed and better able to concentrate.

Try to arrange your life so that you are not always fighting time. Plan ahead so that as far as possible you have time allocated for certain jobs, always allowing thirty per cent longer than you think it is going to take. It will probably take all of that, but if you find you have overestimated the time you can give yourself the treat of a few extra minutes for relaxing and restoring energy before the next big push.

When large tasks loom ahead it is a good idea to try to break them down into manageable units, again allowing more time than you think is necessary for each section. Do resist the temptation to cram your life so full of activity that you are always struggling to keep up so that you do not miss anything. Remember the peace and harmony of the single-food meal? It is worth while applying this principle to our various activities, training ourselves fully to enjoy one thing at a time.

When difficult tasks, difficult decisions, difficult interviews or letters lie ahead, try to arrange to deal with these at the time of day when you know your energy level to be at its peak. Also whenever possible, try to work within your own moods. If suddenly you feel the surge of energy which will enable you to clear out your desk, tackle an overgrown part of the garden, spring clean the cupboard under the stairs – grasp the mood and get started. The impetus to do such tasks is all too fleeting. You will probably find yourself much more involved than you anticipated but what satisfaction when the task is done! You may be tired, even worn out, but how well you will sleep because of this sense of achievement.

Often when we sleep restlessly, cannot sleep at all, or wake in the early hours after a short period of not very refreshing slumber, it is because of some inner tension due to unfinished tasks nagging at the subconscious mind.

How blessed are those like Winston Churchill who are able

to take a short refreshing nap whenever the opportunity occurs and wake up refreshed for the next stint of activity! Unfortunately in days of constant mental stimulation and as life's pace increases, sleep, for many people, is tantalisingly evasive; rather like a beloved but independent cat, who resists every attempt at persuasion, but climbs comfortably into your lap as soon as you are really occupied with some other interest.

Then the *quality* of our sleep seems so variable. Sometimes we sink on to the pillow, find blissful unconsciousness for several hours and awaken with the feeling that we have been in some happy place but cannot remember a thing about it, and that happy peaceful feeling even pervades the day to make us more impervious than usual to the assaults of physical life. At other times, although we may lose physical consciousness, we seem to stay entangled in a web of worry and tension and wake up almost as tired as when we went to bed. The body is to some extent rested, but the mind feels as weary as ever.

Why does the quality of our sleep vary so much? What is the secret of that complete release and refreshment of body and soul which we all need? The number of hours spent in sleep seems less important than its quality when it comes, and the amount needed varies according to the temperament and physical metabolism of the individual. It is sad that in spite of much interesting research into the nature and quality of sleep during recent years, so many people still have to rely on sleeping pills to find the blessed relief of a few hours of unconsciousness. Our deep sympathy goes out to readers who are thus afflicted, and we hope that it is a phase which will soon pass. There are herbal and homeopathic remedies to help this condition, which are not habit-forming like allopathic drugs; and any good health store or chemist stocking homeopathic remedies should be able to suggest alternative treatment – but the transition period between the two different types of treatment will probably require a degree of stoicism and a conscientious effort *really* to practise deep relaxation.

Occasionally people write to me complaining of peculiar dreams or psychic experiences at night. Often these 'experiences' are just the result of some physical discomfort such as being too hot, too cold, bedclothes too heavy, pillow too low or not comfortably placed – or merely indigestion. Any of these can result in a disturbance of the psychic flow which prevents the etheric body from easily becoming free of the physical. This disturbance can be accentuated if we fall asleep with the head tilted back and the chin jutting out. The back of the head and the neck is an important point for the psychic flow. When the soul withdraws from the body in sleep (as at death) it emerges through the top of the head. One can see therefore why the relaxation exercise with the head on a book can be so helpful before retiring. It is so important to have the head in a comfortable position, with the back of the neck well-stretched rather like that of the foetus in the womb. This position has been fully described in previous chapters. Regular practice of the small movements will help to form a habit of holding the head in the correct position almost unconsciously, but remember that these movements must be practised as much with the mind as with the body: that is, give the mental direction; clearly think and see what you want the particular part of the body to do; then relax to the power of the spirit within and let go. This habit of conscious thought followed by a complete surrender to the inner power can bring surprising harmony and peace to mind and body.

Now with regard to the quality of sleep, we have to realise that there are different levels of consciousness, and that we must train ourselves to relax and let go at each level to find complete release of the soul-body. A period of really deep and refreshing unconsciousness will then come more easily.

At the physical level it is important to make sure that our bed is as comfortable as conditions allow. A good piece of board under the mattress will ensure a firm base to support the spine and allow it to stretch and relax properly (hardboard such as Weyroc can be cut to measure by a local do-it-yourself shop or timber merchant). People vary greatly in their ideas of pillow comfort, but to start the night it is a good idea to lie on your back with the pillow arranged to support the back of your head, rather as the book does in the breathing technique in chapter three.

As a further, beneficial exercise for loosening the shoulders, continue to lie in the *savasana* position with your pillow taking the place of the book shown in the photographs. Raise the right hand onto the right shoulder and stretch the elbow up and up and backward so that you feel the pull right across your shoulder and down your back. Hold, then relax and let

7   Stretching the shoulder

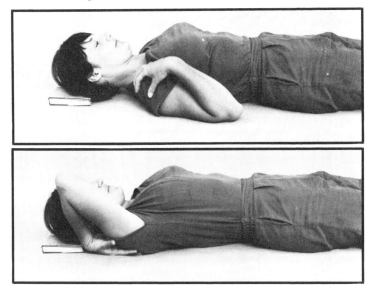

go. Do the same with the left arm. Feel the stretch all the way down your shoulder and back; hold, then relax and let go. You will probably find it helpful to do this shoulder-stretching two or three times, breathing in as you lift your arm: not one long break but perhaps three short ones, lifting the elbow a little higher and further back each time. Now return your hands to your sides and relax.

Mind and emotion can be diverted from daily cares by reading some book which gently holds the interest without stirring up too much reaction – not necessarily a book of any religious nature, but one which turns the mind to pleasant thoughts and pictures.

Helpful also is a warm drink, either some herbal concoction such as lemon balm, or a glass of fortified milk (i.e. dried milk made to almost double strength) with a tea-spoonful of honey. The dietician Gayelord Hauser recom-mends fortified milk not with honey but with a calcium plus vitamin D tablet. Personally I prefer the honey, in spite of its being a miscombination of foods!

The Bach Remedies can be extraordinarily effective in bringing about a more harmonious mental state if you can assess the right one to use. The beauty of them is that even if they are not the right ones they do no harm – but the right ones can be magical. To prescribe them adequately one needs understanding: perception of the *real* cause of the tension and disquiet.

Try to clear the nostrils so that you can breathe freely through your nose, then lie comfortably on your back and for a few minutes just be aware of your breathing. Focus your attention down in the heart – with practice this will soon become easy and habitual.

Feel that with every breath you are becoming part of the eternal rhythms of nature, in tune with the Divine Mother of all form.

Take your mind gently to your jaw-line, and next time

you breathe out drop your lower jaw with a great big sigh. Relax the jaw down and down, and you will soon find yourself giving a deep satisfying yawn. Repeat the process. Once you have started you will probably find yourself yawning several times – a wonderfully relaxing movement for face, throat and indeed all the upper part of the body.

Repeat the quiet peaceful breathing. Now methodically stretch and tense each part of your body in turn – stretch and/or tense, hold, then let go completely: 1) Toes, feet, insteps; 2) Calves and ankles; 3) Thighs and buttocks; 4) Stomach and waist; 5) Lungs and shoulders (another good sigh, then shrug the shoulders up to your ears; tense them and let go completely; bring them down and down); 6) Hands and arms, then fists; 7) Neck, by pulling in the chin and pulling up the top of the head – let go and relax; 8) Teeth and jaws; 9) Eyes: screw up the eye-sockets tightly – hold – relax the eyeballs, look down – right down towards the heart; 10) Face: frown hard – hold – then relax the skin of the face and scalp. Now once again focus your thoughts down in your heart-centre as you resume your quiet peaceful breathing. If your bedding gives just the right degree of warmth, you may well find that sleep has overtaken you even before you reach this stage. You will probably just roll over into your habitual sleep position and know no more. Otherwise continue to focus your thoughts in the heart, and on your breathing; don't try to take great deep breaths, but watch yourself establishing a gentle even rhythm which will gradually become deeper and slower. Try to feel that above you, pouring its light upon you, is a shining Star. With every breath, feel that your body is being filled with light; the light is melting away all the dark tangles of worry and frustration. You are washed clean in the light. Your body is becoming peaceful and easy; your mind and soul are being healed, comforted, blessed by the beautiful light of the Star shining above you. You may even begin to feel aware of the comforting peace and protection of your guardian angel, upholding you in wings of light.

With practice, you will find yourself becoming so absorbed in the Star, so peaceful and illumined, that almost automatically you will let go of the everyday problems which harass the lower mental and emotional bodies. The real you will be free to rise into the higher world, to temples of healing and wisdom, and to your beautiful home in the heaven world where the evanescent problems of the earth life become insignificant against the background of eternal verities. Until you have trained yourself in this discipline of mind and emotions, you will undoubtedly find that the lower mind keeps reasserting itself, especially if you are in the throes of an emotional disturbance. The waves of hurt, resentment and shock keep returning and churning round your mind like a record which has stuck. This is a case for prayer – for an effort of divine will from deep within the soul. Each time it happens, firmly turn your thoughts to the shining Star, and quietly concentrate on breathing in the light. This is the time also to make any affirmations which you want to impress on the subconscious self, and which will help you to come closer to your own ideals of health and behaviour in daily life.

All your mental and emotional disquiets *can* be shaken off. They are all to do with the lesser self, evanescent, fleeting in comparison with the strength and beauty of your real eternal self. They are all just incidents in the long, long path of the soul. Very firmly rise out of all the mental, emotional clutter – yes, even deep sorrow – rise into the shining Star of your real eternal self. Those beautiful rays of light shining down on you are your own Jacob's ladder, down which angels come to minister to your battered soul.

Think of any of the grand old words from your favourite psalms: *The Lord is my shepherd, I shall not want; I will lift up mine eyes unto the hills, from whence cometh my help; They that wait upon the Lord shall renew their strength.* If you find inspiration from the thought, mentally climb to the mountain top, into the rising Sun; focus your thoughts on this. It may be a rough hard climb, but see all your troubles and anxieties as the rocks and boulders, the rough scree over which your spirit clambers with courage and determination, strengthened by the glorious rays of the rising Sun. YOU are rising right out of them into the world of light – into the golden world of God.

Or if you find the thought of the wideness of the sea helpful, deliberately stand back and view your troubles, sorrows and anxieties as a turbulent tossing sea; now rise above the tossing waves and walk on a path of light into the heart of the Sun. See the Sun shining across the water and with all the strength of your spirit rise out of the turbulence and go towards it. The angels of the Sun will help you to set your feet on the path of light. As you walk lightly on the waters all the turbulence dies down and you are coming into the golden world of God – your true home.

Maybe you would find it easier to spread your wings, like Jonathan Livingston Seagull, to rise high above the clouds; leaving all conflicts, controversies and confusions of the little self far behind. See them as thick patches of cloud, while you – the real you – are soaring on the wings of your eternal spirit right up, up, up into the heart of the Sun, with the sure protection of your own guardian angel guiding you safely to your heavenly destination.

Or perhaps your garden is your joy and delight. So let the will of your innermost spirit, the shining flame, withdraw your attention from all the problems of the present day of life. Focus all your thoughts on that tiny clear flame, and think of it as the divine, golden seed shining in the dark earth. Feel the rays of the Sun shining down deep into the earth, awakening the seed to vibrant life. Feel it growing – roots reaching down, shoots rising up towards the light –

opening out leaves, buds, petals to the warmth and glory of the Sun. Be aware of the roots spreading down in the dark earth, drawing strength, nourishment to feed the growing plant: drawing nourishment from all those problems and sorrows which the little self is grappling with in everyday life, but which you have left where they belong, deep in the earth; so that when your spirit awakens to full consciousness it is like the rose blooming in the infinite and eternal garden.

This sense of the unchanging eternal life from which we have come and to which we can return at will is deeply restoring and refreshing. It enables us to view our present problems and sorrows in proper perspective. Learning deliberately to withdraw into this inner, eternal world is a vital key to serenity and health; and even if sleep still proves evasive, this deep relaxation will bring refreshment of spirit.

8

LIVING IN HARMONY

NOTHING IN NATURE ever stands still; either it must grow and develop, or, as soon as it looks like becoming static, it begins to decay and disintegrate. We see this process at work not only in plants and animals but even in the earth itself, for its rocks and stones are, in course of time, reduced to dust by interaction of the elements, the dust being then re-formed into fresh rocks. In the mineral kingdom these transitions take aeons of time to complete. The same law is inexorably at work in the human body, composed as it is of millions of tiny life-cells and governed by a constant cycle of growth and decay. Old and outworn cells die and are (or should be) eliminated from the system while new ones form to take their place. So steady and thorough is this process that over a period of about seven years the whole body is said to be renewed.

The quality of this re-creation depends on the quality of a similar re-creation taking place in man's subtler bodies. The physical, as we said, is but the densest of a number of bodies, all of which are vehicles of expression. Every thought contributes to the formation of the mental body; every emotional response goes towards the formation of the emotional body. In other words, the mental and emotional bodies are created of individual thought-cells and individual 'feeling' cells, in the same way as physical bodies are created of physical cells. These subtler bodies permeate the physical body as salt dissolved in water, or as water permeates a sponge.

Normal human life should follow mother earth in a harmonious cycle of birth, growth, maturity, and then a sweet

130

and peaceful passing onwards to a period of refreshment in the world beyond, before rebirth (or reincarnation). White Eagle tells us that in the Golden Age towards which earth's humanity is now working there will be no disease, no serious degeneration of the physical body even up to the time of death. Man will no longer be afflicted by disease when he learns to live in tune with God. As it is, in youth, the spring-time of life, the life-forces steadily increase in power and decidedly over-balance the decay or negative forces. Because creative forces in the young body can use up what would otherwise have to be eliminated, children can digest and indeed need an amount of heat and energy-giving foods such as would quickly cause discomfort in an adult. At maturity, the life- and decay-forces are balanced; but towards the winter of life the decay-forces begin to predominate as the immortal spirit seeks its freedom. At present few people understand this conception of life; therefore they do not live as long, or as healthy lives as they could, nor is their passing as peaceful and harmonious as it should be. The ancient Red Indians were very long-lived, and except for some waning of the physical energies of youth, their faculties were said to be as good in age as at their prime.

The ability to retain both mental and physical health to the end of our days depends to a large extent upon our ability to live in harmony with the law of change. Physical well-being is not attained merely by superficial treatment of the outermost vehicle. There must be a vital activity in the subtler bodies which are of finer and more malleable substance, vibrating at a quicker rate, but nevertheless subject to the same laws as the physical. Old, unwanted thought- and emotion-cells must be eliminated and new healthy cells formed to take their place. In the same way that congestion and constipation in the physical system causes heaviness and listlessness, so congestion in the subtler bodies can produce a similar effect there.

A constant rhythm of decay, elimination and re-growth takes place. In maintaining health consciously we must learn to co-operate with the dual life-streams – positive and negative, growth and decay, life and death – and by power of spirit, the Son of God within, learn to balance them. When the spirit is able to control the life-forces within its being, so that the rate at which new life-cells are produced and decaying cells eliminated is evenly balanced, the age-long secret of eternal youth will have been discovered.

Our first task then is gradually to create thought- and emotion-habits which are whole ('holy' or 'healthy'). How few of us accept tranquilly circumstances which threaten to break up existing conditions of life, recognising their advent as a symbol of the eternal progress and change which should take place in all healthy lives! We cling to material possessions, love, health or life itself, and all the things we find familiar and dear. We fear loss of prestige, honour, freedom or personal beliefs and prejudices. This attitude is natural, and belongs to the lower self which strives to chain us down. It is due to lack of understanding and vision, lack of discrimination between the real and the unreal. By clinging to conditions, mental, emotional or physical, which are outworn, we cause the dead thought- and emotion-cells to clog the subtler bodies, which are then unable to be renewed by the cosmic life-force. Consequently we feel tired and depressed, vitality is lowered, the physical body sags and we become prey to infection.

Fear, with its companions worry and depression, is the most powerful enemy of health. Between them, they hold up the flow of the life-force and break the rhythm of the various bodies, causing congestion and disease.

To overcome this weakness of the lower self, look diligently and constantly for the good (or the God) in every circumstance and condition, and know with a sure faith that all things are working together for good. This may sound simple and childlike but it covers a deep truth. We have only to observe the manifestations of God in nature to realise the unconquerable beauty and vigour of life. Year after year winter destroys that which summer has brought forth; yet year after year the same plants produce flowers identical to blooms of the previous seasons. Man can do his worst, but given the slightest chance, life in the earth renews itself. In human nature at its best we see the same unconquerable spirit, persevering, enduring, overcoming and rebuilding. This indomitable spirit in nature and in man is God. All the beauty of life – love, kindliness, courage, patience, all that makes us deeply joyous – is divine essence. It does not matter if the forms created are destroyed, for resurrection and progress are eternal. Nothing which is real, which is of the divine, can be taken from us. By meditating deeply on this truth, and keeping our eyes open to it, we may see its universal manifestation. Watch the breaking down of outworn forms and note that even as the old is decaying, springs of life, deep within the root of the plant, prepare for the vigorous putting-forth which is to come. Observe the tiny buds, nestling at the base of the withering leaves each autumn, for they are indeed a symbol of that life, which is unconquerable.

Watching this law at work in nature, we begin to realise its functioning also in every aspect of human life. It helps us to find faith and the inner knowledge that whatever happens is good and progressive. No power on earth can destroy the source of life, within the heart, from which springs all joy, creativity and accomplishment.

Whatever the future may bring we can look forward with tranquillity of spirit, confident that 'winter has its own secret joy, for it holds spring in its heart'.

Never cling to that which must pass, but always look forward; be interested in the trend of events and follow with hope and courage wherever the stream of life leads.

White Eagle's teachings concerning reincarnation and karma can be a real help and inspiration as we struggle with the innumerable problems of daily life. The first blessing of this teaching, once we have taken it to heart, is the increasing realisation that this physical life of every day is only a small section of the eternal path of progress which lies both behind and before us. Without this knowledge it is very easy to sink in a sense of hopelessness, futility, weariness and frustration when circumstances seem to be all against us. We set our minds on a certain objective, something that we want desperately to achieve or attain, and meet innumerable and insuperable obstacles. Without the knowledge of the laws of reincarnation and karma we can so easily wear ourselves out trying to force situations which resist all our efforts.

Once we really digest this knowledge we begin to accept the fact that all the difficulties that face us – difficulties of temperament, family conflict, frustration in work, disappointment in love and friendship, heartbreak over children – all these are the result of causes we have set in motion further back on life's journey. They come to us in this day of life because deep within, in the heart-mind, we know that somehow now we shall find the strength to cope with the situation, to repay the debt owed to the particular soul who is the cause of our sorrow or resentment; to find somehow the tenacity of purpose to 'keep on keeping on' in what seems to be an impossible situation; the courage perhaps to go forward bravely on a path of service, the end of which we only dimly perceive, but to which we feel a deep spiritual commitment.

During our times of quiet prayer and attunement, when we look towards our own Pole Star, we can receive the true guidance of the spirit. It has become a great temptation to rush about to counsellors: to seek advice from many sources, and often to finish in a greater state of confusion than ever. In practical affairs it is sensible where possible to seek the advice of the expert, but in matters affecting our personal relationships, our deep commitments, there is nothing so helpful as what we may call prayer, the source of inspiration of saints and seers through the ages. By this we do not mean the prayer of words, 'Please God, give me what I want; make so-and-so do what I want; help me to achieve what I want'. When White Eagle speaks of prayer, he means a withdrawal from all the claims of the outer life; a putting-aside of all personal desires, ambitions, fears; a conscious withdrawal into a still sanctuary within the innermost being; kneeling before the white altar and watching the clear flame; becoming one with the flame until the whole being seems to be a pillar of light and aspiration. Then from the heart of the flame arises the prayer, 'Father, not my will but Thine'; 'Please show me the way'.

Prayer such as this never goes unanswered. The guide of the spirit will draw very close and a light will shine on the way ahead. The path indicated is often hard. It may well not fit in with what our desire-nature wants, but if we have the strength and courage to follow that path it will lead always to a beautiful and harmonious outworking of the apparently impossible situation. Over nearly fifty years' experience in the work of the White Eagle Lodge, I have witnessed so many lives being changed, so many apparently hopeless situations beautifully resolved, so many people coming through periods of intense suffering on the physical, mental or emotional plane to reach a stage of happiness and serenity where from being patients they become healers.

Just as the ancient astrologers subdivided each day into planetary periods, planetary hours, so the 'day of life' – one human incarnation – can be similarly divided into its planetary periods (like Shakespeare's 'seven ages of man'). These fall in exactly the same order as the diurnal divisions described in my book *Planetary Harmonies* (White Eagle Publishing Trust, 1980).

The Period of the Moon

The first of these periods, the first seven years of life, come under the influence of the Moon, the Great Mother of all life. This period starts with the moment of conception, when the magnetism of the Moon absorbs and draws together all the etheric particles which form the developing body, not only the physical body but what we may call the seed particles of the higher bodies, which will gradually develop as the life unfolds. During the first seven years the child is absorbing all the time, absorbing physical food to promote growth and development but, even more, absorbing the influence of its parents, of the environment which nurtures that soul. This is its karma. Souls who are called upon to endure a distressing, loveless, even tormented childhood have chosen to endure these experiences as an opportunity to gain deeper understanding and compassion, which will eventually flower in some form of selfless service, possibly to some other children similarly affected. For those who have passed through such bitter experiences White Eagle would say, 'Try to forgive'. You have certainly passed through a crucifixion, but if you can open your heart to the warmth of the spiritual Sun you will also know the joy of resurrection and emerge into a happy fulfilment, which hardly seems possible while the mind is frozen in bitterness. Try to let the bitterness melt in the warmth of the Christ Sun, and as you can feel forgiveness healing will flow through every channel of your being.

We would impress on all parents the enormous importance of these first seven years of life, when the child is often more aware of the inner than the outer planes of being. It is during these years that the wise, calm, protective love of the mother and the strength and security of the father is so important.

White Eagle speaks often of the importance of motherhood in the New Age. He says, 'The influence of divine

Mother will irradiate the new age. Motherhood is a beautiful office. There are many advanced egos waiting to incarnate and young parents who are being helped, guided and influenced from the Lodge above. There must be preparation, spiritually, in the souls of the young parents for the coming of those advanced egos. We look to the young . . . *you* may not know their mission, nor that for which they are being prepared; but this you can understand, that your responsibility is to give them spiritual light, spiritual truth, not necessarily by talking to them, but by preserving in the home that which should be sacred to all homes – brotherhood of the spirit, purity, kindness, love and truth'.

The Period of Mercury

Mercury, the planet of the mind, rules the years from the change of teeth to the onset of puberty. During this period the conscious mind begins to assert itself and take precedence over the psychic and emotional receptivity developed by the Moon. This is the age for learning to read, write, calculate, and to some extent to reason. Mercury governs the hands, the tongue and the thinking processes, so this is a time for developing the powers of thought through creative activity with the hands. Mercury develops the longing for movement, for fun and games, for competitive activities both of body and mind. It is a period of life when the energies need to be disciplined and directed by wise teaching methods which awaken the child's interests both in its immediate environment and in gaining skills and developing ideas. The healthy child is full of curiosity, longing to learn and to tackle with interest and enthusiasm whatever task captures the imagination. The development of the imagination will form an important part of the child's training at this stage. This is where drama and acting can be used with advantage to develop the children's interest and help them to enter fully into stories and adventures. At this stage they need plenty of movement and action, competitive games and creative tasks which hold their interest and channel their energy.

Astrologically Mercury is known as a neutral planet, one which, like the Moon, quickly reflects the characteristics of those with more distinctly defined energies. It is not surprising therefore that during this period of their lives children greatly need sensible discipline and direction. They like to know where they are and quickly respond to an adult who can not only arouse their enthusiasm but also teach them how to channel and direct it creatively. They cannot at this stage understand how to discipline themselves, so need the security of a well-structured timetable, quiet, kindly control which protects them from becoming over-excited and over-tired. They also need to feel the security of the religious faith which upholds their parents and teachers. This faith is something which is caught, not taught. Children know instinctively whether adults really believe and understand the precepts which they teach. Children of this age are (as in the first period) extraordinarily good imitators. They will almost unconsciously absorb and imitate the behaviour of adults whom they love and admire. At this stage they will naturally copy the posture and movements of their parents, so it will be particularly helpful when parents can be a living example of that beautiful posture in which the body of light uplifts the physical atoms so that 'the law of levity balances the law of gravity'.

The Period of Venus

The fifteenth to the twenty-second years inclusive come under the rulership of Venus, the planet of love, partnership, human relationships generally – also of art, beauty, finance and possessions. She rules all these matters through her zodiacal signs of Libra and Taurus.

This is the period which mostly covers adolescence, when

the emotional nature begins to awaken with the development of the reproductive organs. With many young people it also coincides with much mental pressure, with examinations in preparation for the career. Conflict between the developing emotions and the increased mental pressure is often difficult for them to balance and resolve. Adolescent people need wise help in learning to cope with their increasing awareness of and longing for the companionship of the opposite sex.

As we have seen, Venus is concerned with finance as well as sex. This is also, then, the time when some young people receive their first pay packets. Unfortunately another aspect of the double influence of Venus is that commercial interests have discovered that anything concerned with sex stimulation is a big money-maker. The pressure upon our young people through an unnatural stimulation of the sex feelings by the commercial interests behind press, radio, television, films and video make this growing-up period far from easy in the Western world.

Some understanding of astrology would, I feel sure, help parents and educationalists to guide their charges wisely during these difficult years of growing-up. Some of the basic principles of Venus are beauty, love, and kindliness; with, at the other end of the scale, laziness, slovenliness and over-indulgence in pleasure. The polar opposite of Venus is Mars, the planet of fire, energy, strength and enthusiasm, also conflict, rebellion and violence. In the horoscope Venus represents young women and Mars young men; and both planets, through their exaltation signs, are closely linked with Saturn, the planet of responsibility, forethought and planning for the future. Much is done at the present time to bring about and to make easy the mental development of young people, but many are left in sad confusion as to how to cope with the awakening emotions which are being artificially stimulated. Even without this stimulation adolescence tends to be a period of stormy emotion, of suffering through the feelings, of intense joy and grief. Sometimes there is great loneliness, self-consciousness; or, at the other end of the scale, too much pleasure-seeking. At this time we may well meet souls with whom we have run up emotional debts in the past, debts which we now have an opportunity to clear, sometimes with much heartache.

In helping young people through this period it seems important to nurture and strengthen their growing appreciation of harmony and beauty, and also the natural idealism of youth. They need opportunities for happy communal life where boys and girls work together at their mutual interests. Every art and craft has its own discipline, as has every form of sport. These activities, which are a source of pleasure and satisfaction, will also help the soul to understand how essential to happy achievement is discipline. Almost subconsciously this will help them in a disciplining of the emotional energies.

Understanding of the physical aspects of sex is essential and ideally should be given towards the end of the Mercurial period when the mind is active and full of curiosity and the emotional nature still fairly quiescent. Then as the emotions develop young people need to be given help in understanding and dealing kindly and wisely with the feelings of the opposite sex. This should be the time for romance and idealism, for the magic of first love, the beauty of springtime. It seems sad that in these materialistic days the bodies of our young girls are often subjected to continuous drugging through the contraceptive pill, so that the awakening sex instincts can be indulged without responsibility.

How many young girls really want this so-called freedom, which purports to be given by 'the Pill'? The influence of Venus awakens in the soul a deep longing for beauty and harmony, for happy partnership and companionship with the opposite sex. Most girls cherish in their hearts an ideal of love and romance, of being wooed and won, cared for and protected by a brave young knight. A law demonstrated throughout nature is for the female of the species to select her chosen mate after he has in some way proved himself and following quite an elaborate courtship. It is natural too for young men at this stage to have an ideal of feminine beauty, however vague and distant this may seem. Falling in love should stimulate all that is best and the highest aspiration in their nature, as they strive to win the affection of their 'lady'. It is a basic fact of human nature that we all appreciate what we have to work hard to win.

The links between Saturn (planet of responsibility, hard work and long-term planning) and Mars and Venus, demonstrates also that no matter what arguments the outer mind produces to justify free sexual indulgence and the satisfaction of the desire-nature, spiritual law, just, perfect and true, teaches that the enjoyment of a sex relationship *always* involves responsibility of the persons concerned both to each other and to any souls that come into incarnation, or try to come into incarnation through that union. In the light of spiritual law, 'free love' does not exist. There is always a price to pay, either happily and willingly in this life, or in sorrow and frustration in some future one, for sexual union always brings a karmic involvement between the two souls.

The sexual emotions of a woman are designed by nature to lead to motherhood. While there are some women in whom this urge is not very strong, there are many who when sexually aroused and deeply in love, become tormented by the longing for a child. It seems perhaps unfair that the fertile years of manhood last so much longer than the woman's child-bearing time which is relatively so short. This reinforces the idea that young women need to be wise and discriminating in their choice of partners and learn how to keep their relationships with young men at a manageable level while they are learning to understand themselves and what they need and are looking for in a life partner. All the great world religions emphasise the need for motherhood to be protected and reverenced. It is perhaps the chief lesson of this period and essential for the health of the race.

Any astrologer knows that the birth horoscope clearly indicates the conditions likely to be experienced with regard to love affairs, marriage and children. We may think that we have a certain amount of choice, but there is probably far less than we realise, for this is an area of life in which we both create and work out much karma. When emotional karma between two souls is ripe to be discharged, the guardian angels will draw them together, often by the strangest chain of circumstances, and they will feel an irresistible attraction. How they cope with this, how they face up to their responsibilities and act towards each other with thoughtful consideration, will determine their relationship at some future time.

During this Venusian period of the life it is helpful to understand that happiness, like money and possessions, has to be earned; and that there is a wide difference between pleasure, which is a passing sensation, and real happiness. Every one in a physical body has frustrations and disappointments to face. It is part of the training of the spirit, the building of the solar body, that we learn to accept the frustrations and to use the opportunities for service which our karma brings.

The Period of the Sun

The fourth planetary period, the age of the Sun, covers the nineteen years from the twenty-second to the forty-first birthdays inclusive. By this time the soul is usually fully incarnated, although there is no hard and fast rule about this, any more than we can exactly gauge the time of the change of teeth, or puberty. It varies with individuals. A soul who has returned to earth with some special mission may even then not be in full command of all the faculties which are necessary for its work, but as a general rule the pattern of the life is beginning to take shape. The Sun astrologically rules the heart, wherein dwells the flame of the spirit, the architect of this day of life.

In the horoscope the Sun is associated with the fifth house, the house of children, love affairs, all matters concerned with pleasure and creativity. During this period the majority of young people will be finding their life partners and creating their own sphere of activity in home and family life, in business or profession, in group activities, social pleasures and hobbies. These nineteen years should be a busy, happy, active period of energetic participation in many responsibilities and interests. Again here we feel the steadying, disciplining power of Saturn, the polar opposite to the Sun, indicating the heavy responsibilities and hard work so often concerned with the upbringing of children.

The outworking of karma in family relationships and in connection with one's children (or parents) is deep and profound. There is no such thing as chance in the family situations which arise; and the more we seek to understand spiritual law and pray for strength and light to fulfil our karmic duties, the more we shall find all the little knots and tangles being dissolved by mutual kindness and affection. In a difficult karmic situation a courageous acceptance of the burden and a willingness to 'go the extra mile', as we are advised in the Sermon on the Mount, will sooner or later result in the joy of increasing spiritual awareness, and in old wounds healed and forgiven, even though the soul may not at first recognise it.

Practice in training the body to maintain its upright posture will strengthen our contact with the mind in the heart and can build into our lives the habit of quiet contemplation. As we begin instinctively to think before making a physical movement, so we also begin to think about our daily routine, to discriminate between important and unimportant matters, and set ourselves priorities of duty and accomplishment which will bring harmony into our daily life. As the body, if undirected by the higher self, will respond to the pull of the earth and slump forward, so in our environment we can either hold ourselves attuned to the Great Architect of the Universe or let matters slide along in a haphazard way and be completely bogged down in the chores of daily existence. Yet people differ much in their ideas of harmonious living. Some need apple-pie order and feel positively tormented in an environment of muddle, while others feel quite suffocated by too much order and routine. Happy-go-lucky, they find the muddle of their environment like a nourishing compost which encourages their creative powers. They are able to concentrate wholly on the project of the moment, ignoring or even feeling comforted by their own familiar clutter.

There is no need for anyone to force themselves into what is, for them, an unnatural pattern of behaviour. Each has their own particular place in the grand scheme; their own special contribution to give to life, but within this wide range of personal preference and ability there can be few people who would not like to become more aware of a wise plan working out in their lives. The mind in the heart is the architect of the small individual life, and in a mysterious way that architect brings us into rapport with the Great Architect of the Universe. If we can train ourselves to become more aware of that still, small voice within we shall be more able to bring into our personal environment the order and beauty of the stars and planets, and to bring the whole life under the direction of the Great Architect. Just as the Pole Star is the centre of the heavens, so each man has his own Pole Star. Even a few moments of concentration each day are sufficient to bring him into alignment with it, and can lead into clear, unbiased thought concerning duties, priorities and values.

Duties and responsibilities obviously have to be accepted

cheerfully as our contribution to life, also as training and discipline of the soul, and often because we deeply love the people to whom we have responsibilities and want to serve them. In thinking about these matters, it is helpful to hold any difficult situation peacefully under the guiding Star and see if any adjustments or improvement is possible. This will often have to be in small ways, small changes of attitude, small kindnesses that ease the path and warm the heart. As we learn to live by the mind in the heart we soon discover how the effort to put just a little extra kindness or happiness into the task sets the heart aglow, our own as well as that of the recipient. It actually stimulates the thymus gland and releases energy and life-force to lighten the task. Dr John Diamond in his researches discovered that even a happy smile produces a surge of energy in the muscles, through the release of the hormone produced by the thymus gland.

The Period of Mars

The fifth age, from the forty-second to the fifty-sixth year inclusive, comes under the rulership of Mars, the polar opposite of Venus, and covers the period of what is commonly known and dreaded as the 'change of life', more recognised in women than men, though it affects both. We may note that the Sun is exalted in the Martian sign of Aries. It is usually during this period that the children are beginning to grow up, giving their parents a little more freedom. However, the child's inevitable desire for freedom often brings battles with the parent, which are associated with the fiery Mars. It is also a time, both with men and women, for forging ahead with their particular interests and ambitions to reach the zenith of their career. In this connection it is interesting that Mars is exalted in Capricorn, the sign of responsibility and ambition, the sign of public service. In its higher aspect Mars is the planet of sacrifice and self-dedication, and during this phase of life much happiness can

145

be gained through devotion to one's chosen form of service to the community. While the children are young, building the family in happiness and security is the first responsibility, but as they 'grow their wings', the experience gained through wrestling with their upbringing can be put to excellent use in wider spheres. During this stage work which is true service – a giving of oneself to life – can be life-giving.

It is also a period when many people come into closer contact with death through the passing of relatives and friends. Early youth often gives us a feeling of immortality, but at this fifth stage most of us begin to be aware that although we feel just the same inside, the physical body is showing signs of wear.

Obviously we need to conserve energy and it is essential to plan for ourselves a certain period each day for quiet when we know that we shall be undisturbed for at least half an hour. Even the busiest person should be able to organise this time, which should be used for conscious relaxation, quiet deep-breathing (see chapter two) and being still under the Star. Most of the time the mind should be held quite still, just revelling in and absorbing the peace of this contact with the divine self, but regularly once a week it is a good idea to use the time for an assessment. Keep a notebook. Think about the week which has passed. Are there areas of your life which would perhaps flow more harmoniously if differently arranged?

Few of us will be able to make big changes because by this time most of life seems to fall into a pattern conditioned by what has gone before. When we start to assess even the small details of our daily routine we soon realise how much we are all tied by factors that in some way we have created in the past. We have involved ourselves in certain responsibilities and duties which have to be met; but at the same time we have probably collected quite a lot of clutter, clutter which

146

impedes our minds, our homes and our activities. This is where the weekly period of quiet assessment can be so helpful. (For an elaboration of this, see again my book *Planetary Harmonies*, p. 64, about 'the day of Saturn'.)

Most of us in our minds have many jobs lined up 'to be done some time' which add to the tension of our lives. Just as we hoard old clothes, odd items that 'may come in useful', we hold in our minds odd preconceptions that we have never thought through and which become prejudices, and most of us also hoard this collection of 'things we mean to do'. On our assessment day it is quite a good idea (some time when we feel fresh after a holiday, or when the mood takes us), to list these various mental pieces of clutter and see if it is possible to have a spring clean. In tackling this kind of mental clutter, particularly when it concerns things one would like to accomplish at some time, it is helpful to view the whole situation in the light of eternity, and to establish the thought that this life is only one short day's journey in eternity. There are obviously priorities. There are ambitions which we realise can never be achieved today; but there really is tomorrow (i.e. another incarnation or day of life), indeed many tomorrows, and all the things that we really want to accomplish, all that the real self, the architect, wants to accomplish, *will* be achieved at some time. Meanwhile let us clear away impractical ideas and ambitions, relax the unconscious tensions, so that we have more energy to make the most of today's opportunities.

Whenever it is possible, several times during the day's work, try to stop for a few moments, relax, and just contemplate some object of beauty, or even the thought-picture of beauty. At the same time think of your physical posture. Are your shoulders relaxing down, is the back of your neck stretching and the head poised? Can you for a moment stand against a wall and feel the line of light from your Star? It may be only a moment's pause to listen to the song of a bird, to breathe in the perfume of a flower or think of the words of a poem, but it will bring a release of divine energy and you will return to your task refreshed. We all need the soul-restoring power of beauty in some form, the form which most appeals to us individually. For many people beautiful sound is most effective. It can be music, natural sounds such as running water, wind in the trees, birdsong or even the crackle of a roaring flame, or it may be colour, or form. Let the mind dwell on beauty, for this builds and strengthens our contact with the divine self. It brings attunement with the Great Architect, creator of all beauty, and restores body and soul.

The Period of Jupiter

The sixth stage, the age of Jupiter, is said to last for twelve years, from the fifty-seventh to the sixty-eighth year inclusive. Jupiter is the planet of the higher mind. White Eagle often explained to patients who came to him for help that the change of life is not only a physical experience. It is also a time of change in the soul, in that the energies are being transferred from the lower centres, involved with reproduction and with finding worldly success, to the three higher chakras which open up the awareness of the spiritual worlds of man's being. During this period, especially now that retirement comes earlier, there should be increasing leisure for contemplation, for the enjoyment of travel, of peaceful hobbies, of philosophical study.

With the prospect of old age there must inevitably come a desire to understand more fully the mysteries of life and death. It is important for every soul who would enjoy a serene and happy old age to seek and find during this period a faith which will sustain them and a knowledge of how to prepare themselves for that initiation which comes to everyone, death. The joy of White Eagle's teaching is that it gives the reassurance and comfort of a sure knowledge that death is but the shedding of an outer garment, like taking off an outdoor coat when the sun grows too bright and hot for it to be worn. The knowledge that birth is not the beginning, nor death the end, but that both are incidents on the eternal journey to the golden world of God, is surely a comfort to those who know that the end of one day's journey is in sight. In the White Eagle healing work we are also shown a way in which we can learn to rise out of the physical consciousness, and even while imprisoned in the body be active in service in the world of light, which can become very real.

This training of mind and soul can be especially comforting when we lose friends and loved ones, through death of the physical body, for during our periods of spiritual service they can draw very close to work with us, in their bodies of light. In this healing work we too are learning to function consciously at the higher level, and it is possible to find a very true and sweet soul-communion with the one in spirit. Part of the purpose of their 'going ahead' is to help their close loved ones to gain a fuller comprehension of the truth and beauty of this form of communion – a soul-unity which can be deeply satisfying. Thus truly, truly, we learn to know the meaning of 'the Comforter'.

The Period of Saturn

The final stage of the journey, from the sixty-ninth year onwards, comes under the influence of Saturn, the planet of hard work, responsibility and limitation, and what should be the serenity of old age. It may perhaps be comforting to souls who throughout their lives have felt the frustrations of Saturnian responsibilities, perhaps through having to care for elderly relatives, or working long and hard for some good cause with poor remuneration – comforting, to know that during this period of the life Saturn usually brings in some compensation and reward. For souls strongly under the ray of Saturn this latter part of life is often the best part – a

149

period of serene happiness and satisfaction.

One of the symbols of Saturn is the bridge. During this period of the life we should be learning to build the bridge between the two worlds. One of the ways in which we can be trained for this is in spiritual service through the direction of good, positive thought, such as in the absent healing work of White Eagle. At this age our minds should be steadied so that we can work quite powerfully on the inner planes; and the more we can learn to focus on the mind in the heart, that eternal flame which will illumine the path ahead, the more we shall be prepared easily to cross the bridge into the world of light when the call comes. Even to the spiritually awakened the thought of approaching death can be alarming, however strong their faith, for at this time the body-elemental, the animal self, is clinging very hard to the mortal life, while the shining spirit finds it increasingly difficult to hold the body-elemental in control.

Extreme old age can be a very difficult time, a real test of patience, endurance and faith. It is at this time that one realises so deeply the power love has, to sustain and uphold the soul both of the elderly person and the relatives. During the final and often difficult stage before the soul's passing into the light, warm human love deepens and expands to build the bridge into the world of light and so enables the angels to make their presence strongly felt. Birth and death are alike in the deep feelings they engender in those that witness them and I am convinced that, just as a baby is not consciously aware of birth into the physical world, the soul passing from the physical life is unconscious of its birth into the world of light. White Eagle has assured us over and over again that always, even in the case of sudden accidental death, preparations have been made to receive the soul in a way that overcomes all shock; and that it will find itself in surroundings that are in no way strange. In the case of someone passing after a long, weary illness, there will surely come a blissful period of sleep followed by a most joyous awakening in a sunlit and dearly familiar garden with loved ones ready with a warm, welcoming embrace.

Such knowledge should take the fear from death but sadly it is often denied to those whose active minds will not let them study the vast amount of evidence both for life after death and for reincarnation, and prefer to push the thought out of their consciousness. Yet, in many souls, the awakening mind in the heart assures them that these things are true. They do not need to read a lot of books or experience psychic phenomena. Deep within they *know*, they remember and bring back the truth from a past life.

This knowledge of the different stages of the unfoldment of the day of life, the knowledge that it is only one short day in the endless years of eternity, should help all of us to accept philosophically the restrictions of our own particular karma. While we can do little about the past, except to deal wisely with the fruits of what we have sown, the future lies in our hands now and it starts in the realm of thought: good thought, creative thought, hopeful thought, loving thought. All around us and within us is the etheric matter to be shaped by thought. All beautiful buildings start as a thought in the mind of the architect; or perhaps first in the mind of the person who engages the architect. Clear, concentrated thought, particularly good, positive thought, will build a harmonious future for every soul. In every life certain karmic debts come up for settlement. They should not be regarded in any way as punishment but as opportunities laying the foundation of future happiness. All responsibilities lovingly met, all frustration and pain bravely endured, all selfless service to the community, is building a golden future of happiness, of even wider opportunities for joyous service and fulfilment.

151

9

SPIRITUAL HEALING AND FAITH

I N THE COMING AQUARIAN AGE the whole of mankind will understand and use the power of thought: will learn how thought shapes the ether at all its different levels of manifestation, and how the etheric mould or pattern created by thought materialises on the physical plane. The clearer and stronger the thought-projection, the more quickly and accurately will it manifest at the physical level.

St John tells us, *No man hath seen God at any time.* The only possible way for the human mind to conceive the Almighty Being, the Creator, is through the Son – the Sun – a shining light, God made manifest. *The light shineth in darkness; and the darkness comprehended it not.* For without darkness, how could we be aware of light? The one is defined by the other. It indicates the duality of creation, positive and negative. Perhaps darkness can be best understood as the basic stuff of creation, the etheric matter waiting to be shaped into form by the divine intelligence. White Eagle sometimes describes it as the brown earth, the unploughed field waiting to be cultivated into a beautiful garden – mother earth.

God created man in His own image, and implanted in us the two aspects, the divine flame and the darkness of the undeveloped ether – the unploughed field. Deep within every man, woman and child lies the God-power to shape by thought the form in which he or she manifests. Furthermore, the life-experience of every one of us is a demonstration of the result of our past thought – thought more than action, for thought is the seed. From this life-experience we are led gradually to discover how the little human personality can become so attuned to the divine intelligence that all the energies of the Cosmos flow through it harmoniously, to create a unique and perfect body and a beautiful environment in which it can function.

'The Ancients saw and worshipped the Sun as sign and symbol of God, and called upon the spiritual sunlight for strength, health and healing. So let us also call.' These words, repeated constantly in our White Eagle healing groups, help the healers to focus their consciousness and attune their small, separate, human personalities to that glorious, universal shining Being, the Cosmic Christ, the source of all healing: the Master of God-thought who creates and recreates all etheric substance. 'O life that makest all things new.'

All souls must discover this in their own way and at their own time. The moment of awakening is unique to each soul, and something which cannot be hurried. At the given moment the soul sleeping in the darkness will, like Lazarus in the tomb, hear the command of the living Christ, and make the effort to throw off the grave-clothes of materiality. Effort, constant and unremitting, it becomes, after the first euphoria of awakening to the light. For there is so much to learn and to be accomplished on the Path that perhaps it is just as well that the first few steps seem to be 'all sweetness and light'.

John Bunyan's story of *Pilgrim's Progress* is one of the clearest expositions of the spiritual path that has ever been written – an allegory of the awakening of the soul to the awareness of the inner Light and its effect on every aspect of the earthly life. First the trap of Mr Worldly Wiseman, which causes the soul to try to judge the path of the spirit by the standards of the earthly mind and worldly wisdom. But the flame of Christ within is so bright, pure, free and subtle that it cannot at all be encompassed by worldly wisdom. It is too simple and humble, and the path appears too ordinary, the service demanded too prosaic – so the soul is lured by mental excitements, apparently compelling psychic discoveries and proofs and the desire to shine in the eyes of the world.

Inevitably there follows a testing time, which lands the neophyte in that hopeless bog, 'the Slough of Despond'. More often than not it will be some dire physical affliction – illness, tragic bereavement, failure, despair at our own or a loved one's inability to overcome some weakness or addiction, that will force the soul to seek for the Source of strength and comfort. It is generally some form of crucifixion, some denial of all personal hopes and desires, that leads us to the awakening of the light of the spirit, that flame of joy which even after the most devastating period of sorrow, sickness or loss will always spring up again to restore the soul, to bring new and more beautiful growth. It is part of the eternal mystery of life and death that the renewal of joy and beauty, of happiness and fulfilment, always follows even the utmost desolation.

In Europe we had wonderful demonstrations of this amazing healing power of nature when after the most devastating bombing in the Second World War, when spring came there would be flowers and grass springing up all over the scarred landscape. This renewal, which is like the rising sun after a long dark night, happens also in the individual life; it happens in broader terms and longer time-cycles in the life of groups and nations, and it happens in the great time-cycles of the astrological Year. This resurrection, this rising again of the eternal Sun, has been celebrated in religions throughout the ages. In Christianity as in the old Egyptian religion the truth was demonstrated by a Christed man. Jesus and Osiris were both betrayed and their bodies apparently destroyed by the darker forces in human nature, but after a period of quiescence, of being locked in the tomb, the Sun rose within that human body and brought every cell, every physical cell, back into radiant manifestation; with the help, consciously invoked, of the great angels of form and beauty, the angels of the Sun.

Jesus came forth from the tomb having rolled away the stone and waited in the garden for the coming of the disciples. This mystery has to be enacted and re-enacted in every human life. There are darker forces in every one of us, forces of the lower self which betray and destroy the temple which the inner Christ is building. To every one of us the karma we create brings crucifixion, which can take place in body, mind or emotions. We all have to accomplish the complete surrender of some part of ourselves, the death of which will make way for new and more beautiful growth. So, dear friend and reader, if you are going through a period of darkness and devastation when you can apparently see no light at the end of the tunnel, hold fast to the enduring thought that the little flame of Christ still shines in the darkness. Meditate on that simple little flame and worship the eternal light which you know will never fail. Give yourself completely to that light and wait patiently. As you do this you will feel the loving hand of brotherhood from those in the world of light, who understand exactly what you are going through. They strengthen the flame in your heart with their love and give you courage to keep on, with the assurance that even *your* crucifixion will end with a glorious resurrection. For at the appointed time the Christ within you rises to push away the stone from the tomb and angels lead you forth into the spring garden, the garden of the rising sun.

The place where we all eventually have to start is within our own physical body, the one material possession that is peculiarly our own – the gift of our parents and forbears; a gift inextricably bound up with their karma and our own. For the blood which flows in our veins is closely and mysteriously linked with the flame – the life-spirit – in the heart. Family karma is a deep and profound spiritual mystery, which one day enlightened scientists of the Aquarian Age will be studying, when the laws of reincarnation and karma are universally understood and accepted.

It is often at this stage that we are led in some strange way to a centre of spiritual healing. At the White Eagle Lodge we have heard through the years, and are still constantly hearing, amazing stories of how souls in dire need are led to pick up a White Eagle book, notice an advertisement, or meet a White Eagle member. We have long since come to believe that there exists a most efficient scanning system in the Healing Temple in the inner world, and a most perfect organisation for rescuing souls in distress and leading to the right teacher those who are ready to progress in their spiritual unfoldment. Over the years there have been so many examples in our work which are evidence of this, and which convince us of the truth and beauty of White Eagle's words; giving us an assurance that if we try simply and earnestly to follow the path he so clearly unfolds, no matter what life brings by virtue of our karma, the wonderful and unfailing help of our dear shining brethren in the world of light will companion us in our troubles and help us over all the rough places.

Many people who ask for spiritual healing are under the impression that all they have to do is to sit back and let the healers in spirit do the work; that if they have sufficient faith, they will be cured. This is undoubtedly true, but real faith, the magic which can work miracles, is quite different from the rather lukewarm hope with which the majority of people approach the spiritual healer.

White Eagle has defined faith as an inward knowing, an inner conviction of truth; it is born of knowledge and experience, but not necessarily knowledge and experience gained in this present incarnation. Many people, when asked how they came to accept certain spiritual truths, will say, 'I just knew somehow. I didn't need any proof'.

Real faith is a potent factor in spiritual healing. Some people are so rich in this quality that not only are they themselves exceptionally responsive to the healing power, but they seem able to channel that power to others on whose behalf they seek healing. They never doubt that once they have brought their friends to White Eagle for healing, everything will be all right, and time after time it is. Those blessed with such childlike confidence in the power of the spirit are found among all kinds of people, some of the finest subjects being those with highly trained minds, who yet retain a humility of spirit which tells them that human knowledge, however extensive, is but a fragment of the whole mystery of life. They bow in reverence before the Great Architect of the Universe and are aware in their hearts of the power of God, which permeates every atom, to heal, restore, renew. Their faith, like that of the saints of old, has been won through tribulation and becomes a source of strength and healing to others.

Most people, however, still have to fight for faith, wrestling with giants of doubt, despair, pain and weariness. 'Lord, I believe; help Thou my unbelief', is the cry of so many who ask for spiritual healing, often after hearing a damning medical verdict. Trained from childhood to use their reason, to doubt, analyse and dissect, to believe nothing unless it be proven, an instinctive childlike faith in the Great Healer seems impossibly difficult for them. Yet to believe implicitly in His presence, in imagination to feel His touch, is to open the door to glorious life-giving power.

It is difficult, in the face of physical pain and weariness, to hold fast to a positive image, for all the forces of gravity conspire to hold the spirit chained in matter, like a seed or bulb locked in frost-bound soil. Only knowledge and experience gives us faith during the long cold winter that the spring flowers are there in embryo, only waiting for the strength and warmth of the sun to call them forth. Similarly, by knowledge and experience the real self, the shining over-soul of every human being, knows that the warmth and power of the spiritual sun, the Christ, is there all the time, waiting to permeate and dissolve the ice-bound material consciousness in which the human spirit is locked. Until a certain stage of spiritual growth has been reached, it is difficult for this higher, Christ-consciousness to penetrate and control the limited physical brain.

If you are sick, sad, anxious, weary or in constant pain, and find it almost impossible to hold on to faith or even to hope, the first requisite is an earnest childlike prayer for light and understanding. Refuse to surrender to the 'pull of gravity', and pray for help that you may learn first to relax and then to rise in consciousness above the limitations of matter. This will enable the angels of healing to draw close.

In this humble, reverent spirit, start to train your reasonable but limited earthly mind to realise that it is only a very small part of the real you. The real you is a radiant being, perfect in the image of God, which has taken on a physical body in order to learn how to gain mastery over the physical atoms. This shining being, the real you, can at present only manifest in a very small degree through your waking consciousness. It is like someone learning the technique of a musical instrument, able at first to play only simple pieces. With constant practice and effort, however, the real you, the Christ-you, will gradually gain complete mastery of the physical instrument and will sound notes and harmonies you are at present unaware of. In other words, the real you will learn to use cells in the physical brain which now lie dormant, and bring radiant health and capacity for service.

Your limited earthly consciousness must be convinced of the reasonable nature of this concept. Make your earthly mind accept the truth that it is merely an instrument for the real you, and that the awareness conveyed by the five senses is very limited compared with what *you* know and do when free from the physical vehicle in sleep. This will take time and patience, but it is the first step towards that inner conviction which is faith.

Before relaxing into sleep, think about this freer, fuller life of the soul, and try to picture the temple of healing, to which you may be taken to receive the touch of the Great Healer. By so doing, you will gain the co-operation of the subconscious – or perhaps we should say superconscious – mind, so that gradually the shutter which closes when you wake, to cut you off from your higher self, will not be so tightly fixed. You will begin to notice that during the day ideas and impressions will come to you which help you to think more positively. Instead of being all the time tense with anxiety, fear, pain and weariness, you will find moments of peace and a lightening of the load – fleeting moments perhaps, but nevertheless like shafts of sunlight, or the touch of angels' wings, or the gentle hand of the Great Healer on your brow. Train your lower mind to recognise these moments of greater awareness, and to realise that it is gradually coming under the direction of the higher self, the real you.

The story of Jacob's ladder, which was built while he slept, and down which angels came and ministered to him, portrays an eternal truth. Every soul must eventually learn to receive the ministry of angels by building the ladder between heaven and earth; and one of the first steps is to use this creative imagination before drifting into sleep. It will help to bring strength for the battles to come: for make no mistake, that faith which will carry the soul to victory over physical inharmony is not a faint-hearted hope, it is an undaunted strength and courage, won after many a battle with darkness and despair.

'Hold fast to the certainty that Christ within you is king, and can overcome all weakness, all sickness, all inharmony.'

This injunction, part of White Eagle's contact healing service, is worthy of constant repetition, especially when pain and frustration would dominate the earthly consciousness.

But don't be tense and over-enthusiastic in your efforts to demonstrate the supremacy of the Christ within – fierce fires soon burn themselves out. What is needed is a steady flame of faith, a quiet conviction that the Christ within will manifest the perfection of spirit, of God, through the physical body, gently, slowly, cell by cell, day by day, as you quietly practise the small movements previously described and hourly draw upon the divine strength and energy within – the living flame – the architect of your whole being.

Resist not evil, but overcome evil with good. In other words, concentrate not on *fighting* sickness, pain and frustration, but on building the image of the perfection which the Christ in you will manifest. Do not think in terms of time, because this immediately arouses the natural impatience of the lower mind to cry, 'O Lord, how long?' and to concentrate on the present chaos instead of the perfect image. Quietly, persistently, create – and keep creating – this image of harmony and perfection.

This is not quixotic or unworldly. When an architect wishes to create a beautiful building, he first sees it in his mind. He visualises the finished structure, and then works out the practical details. Then he directs the work of the builders and contractors. If the builders work without the architect, numerous details of the original plan go awry. The Christ self is the architect of the perfect human life, working as one with the Great Architect of the Universe. The Christ in you sees the perfection which will manifest. When you hold the perfect image, ignoring the present chaos, you consciously identify yourself with the Great Architect, enabling Him to direct the builders. You bring your God-will to bear, gently but irresistibly. Besides enabling you to hold fast to the vision beautiful, this God-will will prompt you to deal wisely with the practical details of daily living. It is unreasonable to expect God to work miracles if the normal rules of health are disregarded. Man has to learn to *render therefore unto Caesar the things which are Caesar's*, but when he fulfils the whole obligation and begins also to render unto God the things that are God's, the healing magic surely works.

10

THE HEALING TOUCH

MANY PEOPLE LONG to be able to give healing but do not know how. They have no faith in their own powers and do not realise that it is possible for anyone to become a healing instrument if they will train themselves to focus their thoughts and open their hearts to Christ, the Great Healer.

The true healing power, whether for humans, animals or plants, is love; human love strengthened and illumined by that divine love which can flow through the hands as light – light which restores first the etheric body, where the disease shows as dark patches, and then the physical body. It is possible for anyone to train themselves so to still mind and emotion that their whole being is open to the Christ Sun, which is then directed, with clear, precise thought, to flow through the hands as a ray of light; which then floods the etheric body of the patient, dissolving the disease and stimulating in the heart of the patient the divine flame, the Christ self, which will take command and bring the healing right through into physical manifestation.

This direction of the Christ light focused by the thought of the healer can be as effective at a distance as in healing by touch, or what in the White Eagle Lodge we term 'contact healing'. Indeed there are some patients who are happier not to be touched by human hands and who respond well to absent healing. Others find the healing touch comforting and helpful, and there is no reason why anyone who longs to help in this way should not give a simple form of healing by touch.

162

There are, however, two important rules to observe. The first is to be absolutely sure that the patient is a willing recipient of such treatment. It is a great mistake for the eager spiritual healer in any way to force his ministrations if there is the slightest hesitancy on the part of the patient. For the healing power to flow freely, there must be calm, gentle, understanding love on the part of the healer and a completely happy and relaxed response on the part of the patient.

The second rule is that the healer should be physically fit. With contact healing, inevitably there will be some transference of the physical magnetism of the healer into the etheric body of the patient. An abundance of physical magnetism is often apparent in natural healers who choose to work in the medical profession, or in osteopathy, physiotherapy or the less orthodox healing methods. Any of these dedicated servers almost unconsciously passes on to his patients a vitality and strength which makes the patient immediately feel better for their presence. These professional healers, through their long discipline and training, will convey this strength and confidence to their patients even when they themselves are physically exhausted. They have learned to tap inner reserves which enable them to keep giving as long as they are on duty. On the other hand amateur healers, those who long to be used by the power of the spirit, but are without the discipline of this professional training, should not attempt to give healing unless they have plenty of usable vitality, for it is possible for the would-be healer unconsciously to draw vital force from the patient instead of giving.

I would emphasise that this is *not* the case with absent healing, healing from a distance through the power of prayer. I hope that this will encourage those who, after a lifetime of service, healing and caring for others, now find themselves too old and weary to continue their service on the physical plane. If the desire to serve is still strong it is possible to give really effective spiritual healing even if the healer is confined to bed or chair, for in the soul-world distance is nothing. There is no space, no time; it is all a question of consciousness – God-consciousness. By raising our thoughts, our being, to the Christ Sun and feeling at one with the Great Healer, we can lift the soul of the patient into that wonderful healing presence. The effectiveness of this has been proved literally thousands of times during the nearly fifty years that the White Eagle absent healing has been at work. In fact we believe that to sit as a healer in a White Eagle healing prayer group is an essential part of the training and preparation of those who want to work as contact healers.

Provided then that the patient is happy and receptive and the healer buoyant with vitality, how can contact healing be given? Often all that is required is a gentle drawing-off of the congestion in the etheric body which is causing a blockage in the flow of life-force resulting in pain and disturbance in the physical body. Then with the right hand held lightly and peacefully over the sore spot the healing light is poured in. This treatment can be used for all kinds of minor aches and injuries, especially those in the limbs.

To draw off pain or discomfort, first settle the patient in a comfortable position where you can easily reach the affected part, and suggest that they imagine that they are relaxing in a sunbathe. In all healing work we train ourselves to function not so much in the head as the heart-mind. Breathe quietly and peacefully, focusing all your thought on the Sun, the spiritual Sun behind the physical sun. With every breath feel your heart being filled with the life-force from the Christ Sun. The light courses round your body in the bloodstream and every cell is being filled with light. As the words of the White Eagle absent healing service say, 'We are now become as flames of Thee, golden Light of the heavens, heavenly radiance and illumination.'

Being thus filled with light you should not find it difficult to focus that light through your hands. See your fingers with rays of light streaming through them, like the prongs of a grass-rake which will pass right through the physical atoms of the patient's body to reach and comb away the dark patches of congestion in the etheric body. Very gently, and barely touching the patient, place the fingers of both hands well above the pain or injury and slowly draw them right down the limbs and off at the fingertips or toes. Imagine that your elongated fingers are combing out of the aura some of the shadowy congestion, which you gather up in your curved fingers and draw right down to the end of the fingers or toes, and then flick off, directing it back into the earth. Gently make this drawing-off movement down the limb and off at the fingers and toes quite a number of times, all the while trying to visualise the light pouring from your fingers, combing away and dissolving the shadows, directing them down into the earth. Do this until you feel that the congestion is clear, then very gently and lightly place your right hand over the painful spot, with the left balancing it at the other side of the limb, and peacefully concentrate on the glorious, healing Sun. Feel that the light in your heart-centre is a flame in the heart of the eternal Sun – the Cosmic Christ. Let that pure flame radiate through every cell of your being until you and the patient are enveloped in almost unbelievable brilliance of light.

The more clearly you can hold the concentration, the more freely the healing power will flow through you. With practice you will be able to hold this spiritual contact for several minutes, and may become conscious of a great warmth, even a tingling sensation in your right hand, as if an electric current were pouring through you. Do not struggle to hold it for too long. Quietly and peacefully maintain it for a minute or two, then stop. Mentally ask for the blessing of the Great Spirit, Christ, and pray that the angels of healing will continue the work.

This very simple routine can be most effective with children and animals. Little children who have hurt themselves after a fall often respond quickly, especially if the healer can also find something to divert their interest away from the hurt.

Animals also are remarkably responsive to spiritual healing, far more so than many humans, because they do not put up any mental resistance. So if you desire to heal your own pet, choose a time when the animal is quietly settled in as comfortable a position as possible. Sit beside it where you can easily stroke down the spine gently from head to tail. Again see the rays of light from your fingers going right through the animal's body, combing away the dark shadows of pain and dis-ease and awakening the vital force in the little creature. Unless your animal has actually 'heard the call' of the angel of death he or she will surely respond to the healing.

It is important when you heal that your touch should be very light and gentle, especially if you are healing the head; when a light stroking of the brow with the tips of your fingers, almost the feather-like touch of a butterfly's wing, will surely be the most effective.

Try to realise that you bring healing not so much by your touch as by a calm serenity in your soul, which gives the patient hope and confidence. If you train yourself powerfully to focus your thought on the Christ Sun you will find that with practice you will be able to give beautiful healing with very little fuss. For inexperienced healers, when the pain or disease is situated in the internal organs, it is probably best to direct the healing ray through the throat-centre in the following way.

A good healer can cleanse the whole aura of a patient and direct the healing light to that part of the body which needs help by placing the palm of the right hand at the back of the patient's neck, just where neck and shoulders join. This corresponds to the throat-chakra. It is where most people collect a great deal of strain and tension. When they are worried, overwrought, or fearful, they naturally tense and raise the shoulders, impeding their easy breathing and stopping the free flow of the life-force round the body and the aura. The healer who is able to firmly quieten the outer mind and tune in to the Christ Sun can, by placing the right hand warmly, comfortingly, over the throat-centre at the back of the neck, radiate this healing Christ power right through the aura of the patient. It is helpful to do this with the rhythm of the breathing. As you breathe in, feel that your heart and mind are opening as a flower to absorb the spiritual sunlight. As you breathe out, feel this light pouring through your hands down into the heart of the patient, quickening the Christ light in the heart which in turn fills the bloodstream with light so that with every breath the whole being of the patient is flooded with the Christ radiance and strength.

When you feel that this flow of light is thoroughly established in the rhythm of the breathing, mentally direct a specially bright ray of light to the particular part which is needing help. Again use the rhythm of the breath to become charged with light and then mentally to direct it into the diseased part of the patient's body. You will find that most patients will be much comforted if at the end of this treatment you gently but firmly work your hand round their shoulders in a clockwise direction, giving a good, comforting, warming massage, and finishing with your hand between their shoulderblades to give warmth, strength and comfort to the heart.

This treatment, pouring in the light at the back of the neck in this way, is one which can easily and unobtrusively be given to patients in hospital. It is not always desirable in the conditions of a hospital ward to give obvious spiritual healing, because it could cause embarrassment to the patient and lay them open to unwanted questioning afterwards. Healers must remember that their very presence should bring to the patient a feeling of comfort and security. Through the healer's serenity of spirit they should absorb a sense of peace and confidence in that divine power which upholds every life, and respond almost like a relaxed, sleepy child. When the patient is relaxed in this way, through the powerful tranquillity of your spiritual attunement, the healing angels can draw very close to envelop the patient in wings of light and peace. Try to visualise this happening even while you are sitting quietly chatting.

Remember also that the left side is the receiving side; so if you are anxious to give help, and conditions are difficult, sit on the left side of the bed and gently hold the patient's left hand between your two palms, your right palm in contact with the patient's and your left palm enveloping the back of the hand. Again, quietly, on the rhythm of the breath, direct the light through the left hand of the patient, up the arm and right into the heart, whence it flows all round the body.

If you are visiting terminally-ill patients, you should be careful about sitting for too long holding their left hand in this way because you will find it to be a great drain on the vitality. Time the treatment carefully and then carefully move to a different position; or alternatively, do not give the treatment until it is nearly time for you to leave, allowing not more than twenty minutes. Then be sure to wash your hands right up to the elbows in cold water as soon as possible afterwards.

If you feel that you are likely to be drained by psychic links with the patient you should deliberately cut these links and seal the centres at the solar plexus and the back of the neck. Psychic links are like little threads of a spider's web which are formed when there is any kind of emotional link between healer and patient. They possibly arise through a subconscious desire on the part of the patient to cling on to the source of vitality; and, on the part of the healer, through emotional giving. This is not a healthy condition either for healer or patient; it is the undisciplined reaction of the body-elemental of both, the desire-body of both. True healing will raise the patient's spirit above all the turmoil, weakness and weariness of the earthly life and the personality, right into the heart of the golden spiritual Sun. Although healers need to feel sympathy and compassion, they must not allow themselves to be drawn down into the emotional turmoil of the patient's condition; and would be wise to remember how Christ lightly and radiantly walked on the water. They must call upon the Christ, shining through their heart-centre, to reach out a hand to lift the patient above the turmoil, even as Jesus stretched out his hand to Peter, who tried to walk over the water towards him and through fear was sinking. The work of the healer is so to strengthen the Christ self, the solar body of the patient, that it takes command of its own physical atoms, bringing them into harmony.

If the healer becomes emotionally involved with a patient in a less positive way, psychic links, which are not unlike a spider's web, may be formed; and along these links the patient continues to sap the vitality of the healer long after the treatment is over, clinging mentally and emotionally to the source of comfort.

So, after giving a healing treatment always remember to wash the hands under running water (cold or tepid); take two or three sips of cold water; and if you feel that there are psychic links because of your loving sympathy with the patient, hold your hands under the running tap and flick drops of water from your wet hands over the top of your head to the back of your neck and shoulders and imagine a shower of silver light clearing away congestion, cutting any links at the back of the neck. With firm mental direction see the back of the neck sealed with an equal-sided cross of light within a circle of light. You can do the same at the solar

169

plexus. Flick drops of water from the running tap down the front of your body and with both hands make a cutting motion in front of the solar plexus, as if you were brushing away spiders' webs. Again imagine, like a shield in front of the solar plexus, a cross of light encircled by light. Having cut the psychic links which are connected with the lower self and the body-elemental of both of you, for a few moments concentrate wholly on the Christ Sun. With all the strength of your being and in the name of Christ call upon the angels of healing to lift the soul of the patient into the presence of the Great Healer. With childlike faith hand over the whole problem to the Great Healer, then deliberately turn your mind to other matters and pick up the threads of your own life.

For those who are in the sad position either of constantly visiting terminally-ill patients in hospital, or nursing them at home, the above precautions should be carefully observed because in these cases the body-elemental of the patient will be full of fear and as if drowning will instinctively cling to the would-be rescuer, in a way that could cause the latter to feel submerged as well. It is essential for the healer to hold fast to the contact with the Divine Source of strength which will give the ability – the divine wisdom and love – to keep on patiently and faithfully coping with the practical difficulties and helping the patient to rise out of the vortex of fear, desolation, anger, frustration – all the negative emotions which rise up when the soul realises deep within that the time has come to relinquish their hold on earthly concerns.

At the present stage of medical knowledge concerning the effect of drugs on the psyche, many ageing and terminally-sick patients suffer from a soul-disturbance which makes life extraordinarily difficult for those who love them. There are drugs which seem to affect certain of the chakras, exposing the soul to astral and psychic conditions which at times seem to change their whole personality. There is much still to be learned about the etheric body, the body-elemental and the true self, and it often seems that physicians are working in the dark, unaware of the psychic effect of the drugs they prescribe. The personality changes which are so distressing to loving friends and relatives can only be regarded as some difficult karma brought over from the past which is being worked out between the souls involved. It is in cases like this that the healer or the loving relative can give most help by recognising the fact that the uncharacteristic reactions of the patient are almost entirely disconnected from the true self. What is manifesting through the body is the lower aspect of the body-elemental or the earthly personality, which because of drugs or physical deterioration is no longer within the control of the higher self. Sometimes the thread of light between the two is almost non-existent and the body is only being kept alive by the elemental, which does not want to let go and which will draw strength from any source available, more especially from those who are emotionally attached to the patient.

In cases where it is obvious that the higher self has almost entirely withdrawn it may be better for the physical needs of the patient to be met by caring professional nurses rather than by emotionally drained relatives. The relatives will then have more spiritual strength to give through loving, conscientious healing by prayer and during regular visits to the patient. By holding the loved one mentally under the Christ Star, a ladder of light is formed down which the healing angels can come to minister to that soul.

Sometimes an advanced soul appears to be chained to an earthly body for no apparent reason. They are sweet, gentle and loving but apparently quite unaware of what is going on around them. Where such a soul has given devoted service to others during their active life, it may well be that they are holding the link with the body in order that their strong, radiant soul may work among the disquieted souls in the lower astral world, doing a stint of 'rescue work'. In such cases the body-elemental is being maintained at the lowest possible ebb in order that the soul may descend into the underworld for this service.

When there are distressing character-changes, healers can give most help by not allowing themselves to be drawn into emotional conflict with the body-elemental, which needs quiet, kindly and firm discipline; but rather by focusing their thought upon the shining Star of the true self. They should try to visualise a shining light enveloping the patient, a wigwam or cone of light, seeing him/her within this shining circle protected from all shadows and darkness of the astral world. Constantly to see the light shining down into the patient's heart will strengthen the pure flame of the spirit. Even if there seems to be little effect on the physical condition you can be sure that the soul is being healed and restored so that when it is freed from the physical body it will go forward joyously to its new work in the world of light.

Many patients coming to the White Eagle Lodge for healing have been greatly helped by the Bach remedies. A note about the Dr E. Bach Centre is given at the end of this chapter. As their leaflet 'The Bach Flower Remedies', states, 'The system and the Remedies were discovered by a doctor who had practised for over twenty years in London as a Harley Street consultant, bacteriologist and homoeopath. The late Edward Bach, MB, BS, MRCS, LRCP, DPH, gave up his lucrative practice in 1930 to devote his full time to seek energies in the plant world which would restore vitality to the sick, so that the sufferer himself would be able to over-come his worry, his apprehension, etc, and so assist in his own healing . . .

'The remedies used are all prepared from the flowers of wild plants, bushes and trees, and none of them is harmful or habit-forming . . . As the Bach Remedies are benign in their action and can result in no unpleasant reaction, they can be used by anyone. The measure is small – a few drops in a little water.'

These remedies can be surprisingly potent provided that the right one is prescribed. They are designed to balance the moods, feelings and emotions of the patient, and if they do not seem to be effective it is probably because the person prescribing has not correctly assessed the cause of the trouble. When the correct remedy has been prescribed, the change both in mental outlook and in physical health can be almost magical. This simple form of homeopathic treatment combines well with spiritual healing, for both are working at the soul level to heal the real cause of the physical disturbance.

When you are dealing with cases of terminal illness, difficulties of communication arise when the patient either does not know or cannot accept the true nature of their illness. Dealing with this situation needs loving wisdom, gentle, kindly speech and, most of all, a sure faith in the love and care from the world of spirit which is always present at the approach of death. Gentleness is so important. It is never wise to force the patient to accept facts which they cannot yet face. However much spiritual knowledge the soul may have gained, the thought of losing the physical body can be alarming, even terrifying, for at this time the body-elemental, like a child or an animal, clings to what it knows. There may come a time when it is helpful to the patient to know what they have to face, and to discuss it with the healer. To understand the care that is needed when this time comes, you may be helped by following Elisabeth Kübler-Ross's work with the dying and their families (see note at the end of this chapter). But your task as a healer is to convey to your patient the reality of the beautiful heaven world. As White Eagle says in *Spiritual Unfoldment I*, 'Never suggest that a patient is likely to die. Admit no such thing as death. See only creation, ever changing, unfolding life.' It is for you as healer gently, peacefully, with your vision on the eternal

Sun, to help the patient to build the bridge of light into the golden world of God. By directing the patient's vision constantly towards eternal life, where there will come reunion with loved ones, and joyous, satisfying work and interest, healers with sure faith and spiritual knowledge can bring strength and peace to the patient facing the great unknown.

The ancient Egyptians as well as the North American Indians used to look towards the setting sun which, for them, was like a golden arch into the world of light. It is not easy for the soul about to set forth into this golden world to surrender all the interests of the earthly life; but with quiet, serene, loving help from the healer and a steadfast building the bridge of light between the worlds the soul, when the call comes, will be gently taken by the healing angels into the temple of the setting sun, into the golden world of God, where they will gently and peacefully sleep until they are ready to awaken, refreshed and happy, in beautifully familiar surroundings. Often this is a garden with which they have already become familiar in their sleep state; a garden so like a beloved earthly garden that the soul may think that they are still in an earthly body, except that they feel so light and comfortable, so at peace.

From accounts which have been collected of experiences of people who have been clinically dead and then resuscitated, it is quite clear that the after-death state can be truly beautiful for those who have prepared for this by building the bridge of light. For the ordinary person who has tried to live in a kindly, law-abiding fashion, the after-death state will at first be in what Spiritualists call the "summerland", in which conditions are similar to but usually more beautiful than those of earth. It is comforting and helpful always to remember that every life, no matter how exalted or degraded, is in the loving, compassionate care of a guardian angel as well as a wise human teacher. No soul is ever left

174

helpless or comfortless. As soon as a prayer, a cry for help, goes forth from the heart to God, the almighty, all-loving Spirit, a line of light is instantly created, a Jacob's ladder down which the angels of light can come to lift that soul out of darkness and fear into the world of light. But the key to the golden world lies in the human heart. The door has to be opened from this side of the veil. No angel, no loved one in spirit, can do more than look on in sorrow and compassion until through aspiration to God the soul imprisoned in the flesh turns the key and opens the heart to the warmth and comfort of the love and companionship of the heavenly beings who are so close. In the words of the poet, Francis Thompson:

'The angels keep their ancient places:
　　Turn but a stone and start a wing;
'Tis ye, 'tis your estranged faces
　　That miss the many splendoured thing.

'Yea, in the night, my soul, my daughter,
　　Cry – clinging heaven by the hems;
And lo, Christ walking on the water
　　Not of Gennesareth but Thames!'

Gently, patiently, with a serene tranquil spirit and a sure faith, the healer must help in the building of the bridge of light between the two worlds. This has to be done not so much with words as with all the strength of the spirit. Particularly if the patient is a close relative, a loved one being nursed at home, the healer will need to strengthen contact with the mind in the heart, the source of eternal strength and light many times each day. Whenever there is an opportunity to do so practise the Star-breathing for a few moments, firmly withdrawing the mind from practical concerns and focusing entirely on that clear flame of the spirit deep in the heart. Kneel before the flame and pray for strength. Feel the radiant Star from above forming a pyramid of light, a temple of light which protects the flame and enables it to grow in strength and brightness, melting away all the dark shadows of fear, weariness and distress. This light of the spirit will encompass both healer and patient, dispersing all shadows so that the angels of healing can draw close and minister to both.

It is not by chance that souls are drawn together in the relationship of healer and patient. Those who find themselves nursing a sick relative, sometimes in extraordinarily difficult conditions, should take comfort from the knowledge that this is a God-given opportunity both to repay a debt, probably from a past life, and for both the souls involved to learn more about the true nature of divine love and how this can illumine even the darkest places in the valley of shadows.

Truly, the death of the physical body is only an incident compared with the soul-battles that have to be fought as the spirit learns gradually to triumph over the darkness of fear, resentment, hate, frustration – all the negative emotions which are part of our lower selves, the body-elemental. Those who are drawn together in the close relationship of healer and patient in this battle with the shadows can establish such a wonderful link of love and brotherhood that death of the physical body is as nothing. The true communion of spirit which is established as the bridge of light between the two worlds becomes stronger, is indescribably beautiful; so that when death brings release from the physical body, the arisen soul can awaken the consciousness of the loved one left on earth to the glorious happiness of the heaven world.

This is why the loss of a loved one through death of the physical body can be a wonderful blessing rather than a tragedy for those left behind. Though there is the sadness of the physical loss, if those left behind can be brave enough, unselfish enough, to refuse to wallow in it, and with all the strength of their spirit look into the heart of the Sun, into the golden world of God, giving all their love to the one who has been freed, then that bridge of light between the two hearts becomes so strong and bright that true and perfect communion can be established, a communion so real and satisfying that doubts of the earthly mind melt away like icicles in the sunlight.

The symbol of the six-pointed Star helps us to understand how this can happen. The shining flame of the spirit, the true selfless love in the heart of the soul left on earth, is like the upward-pointing triangle, symbolic of the soul aspiring to the heaven world, building the bridge. As soon as this happens the light from above pours down. The soul of the loved one in spirit can draw close, like the downward-pointing triangle. The union of this with the flame in the heart causes the glorious star to blaze forth as the two souls are together raised into the light. At first when this bridge is established there will just be such a feeling of joy, peace and thankfulness filling the heart that there is no need for anything else. It is like a warm, loving embrace which wipes out all thought of separation. Once the bridge has been firmly established experiences will come during meditation of enjoying together the beauty of the infinite and eternal garden in the inner world. The soul freed from the body will be able to help the one left on earth to awaken the higher consciousness; and this will in turn bring increasing wisdom in coping with earthly affairs, and the deep peace which comes from growing faith in that divine Love which encompasses all our lives.

NOTE

The Bach Remedies, and information on how to prescribe them, are available from the Dr E. Bach Centre, Mount Vernon, Sotwell, Wallingford, Oxon OX10 0PZ. You may find there is a more local stockist, and the Dr Bach Centre may have its address.

Dr Kübler-Ross's books are written for the professional involved in care with the dying, but can be read by others also, although you should remember that her particular work is for the trained counsellor and requires great wisdom and discrimination. We recommend *On Death and Dying* (Tavistock, 1969) and *Living with Death and Dying* (Souvenir Press, 1982). White Eagle's book *Sunrise* (White Eagle Publishing Trust, 1958) is for the bereaved and all those afraid of death; and many who have to face terminal illness have found *The Quiet Mind* (available in a large-print edition as well as a pocket-sized one) a source of daily or hourly comfort (White Eagle Publishing Trust, 1972, 1983).

11

THE ANGELS OF COLOUR AND HEALING

THE WHITE EAGLE HEALING work has always involved close co-operation with the angelic lifestream, both in the prayer groups for absent healing, and also in the laying-on of hands. Many times White Eagle has spoken of the work of the angels, and prophesied that in the coming age of Aquarius there will be a growing awareness of how angels and men can co-operate in creating a more beautiful world and a more harmonious civilisation.

Knowledge of the angelic stream of evolution was part of the ancient wisdom. It is a basic concept of all the great religions and forms part of the magical practices of primitive tribes all over the world. As the soul of man has become more deeply immersed in matter, and as the conscious mind has become more active, the conception of the angelic presences has also materialised. Through the centuries of the Piscean age artists have portrayed solid, fleshy angels with birdlike wings. In primitive tribal symbolism angels are also often depicted as winged creatures, either birds or animals, usually portraying some soul-quality which the angel represents – either good or evil – for there are angels both of the positive and the negative life-streams.

How White Eagle describes angels is closer to the eastern *devas*, beings of light in the soul-world, co-workers with the divine Mother, the feminine aspect of creation, the builder and the destroyer of physical form. At present the creative work of the angelic kingdom is only dimly realised by the mind of man; but during the Aquarian Age, as the spiritual awareness of mankind develops, ordinary people will learn how to bring their lives into harmony through conscious co-operation with angels – with their own guardian angel, with the nature spirits in their plants and gardens, and with planetary angels, those great beings concerned with the elements, who subtly permeate the soul-life of humanity (as shown in people's astrological make-up as well as in the physical elements).

Perhaps the greatest difference between the human line of evolution and the angelic is that humans feel emotion whereas the angels work with absolute dispassion in obedience to a divine plan, an infinitely beautiful cosmic design. The guardian angel in charge of each human life holds that life under a ray of light and power which ensures the completion of the design for a particular incarnation. One might almost liken the working of the angelic kingdom to a cosmic computer under the control of the divine mind. Angels and humans need each other, but until the evolution of both reaches a certain stage the co-operation between them is unconscious. However, the quickening of the mind, both the head- and the heart-mind, which will come as the New Age advances, will facilitate this co-operation. White Eagle teaches that it will result in a quickening of the very earth itself and raise the consciousness of all earth's people to a finer, purer level until the veil between the two worlds of man's being is almost non-existent.

In the past, souls who were ready to follow a path of spiritual unfoldment withdrew into mystery schools, monasteries, secret inner brotherhoods, where they received special training and discipline and had to pass many tests before they were given knowledge of how to work with the angels to produce magical results. Now, at the beginning of the Aquarian Age, this knowledge which was so carefully protected and only given after much training and testing is becoming more widespread. There is an ever-increasing interest in psychic phenomena, extra-sensory perception, spiritual healing, magic, witchcraft. In studying all these subjects, we immediately enter the mysterious hidden realm of the inner world, or what was in ancient times termed the 'underworld'. It requires care. We need to understand something of the working of those darker angels, the 'principalities and powers' of which St Paul and mystics and seers have spoken.

The White Eagle teaching, particularly his teaching for healers, is designed to help simple people who earnestly desire to heal and serve others to learn how to invoke the help of the angels of light. The work of a spiritual healing group is like using a terminal of the divine computer, which in a magical way draws to the sufferer angelic help beyond our earthly understanding. The first prayer healing group came into being under White Eagle's direction in 1936; and even then, with inexperienced and unpractised sitters, the results were such that the number of patients grew rapidly from the start through recommendation. This has continued throughout the years so that we are always needing more dedicated workers to meet the ever increasing demand for help. After years of being at the receiving end of multitudinous cries for help and also the feedback from patients I find my faith in the magical power of the spirit to heal to be stronger than ever. At the same time I realise ever more clearly that the healing of a soul is not necessarily the same as the removal of a physical symptom. We have many apparently miraculous results, especially those in which the prayer groups support the skill of the medical profession, to produce effects which the doctors themselves admit are quite beyond their expectations. But, apart from this, spiritual healing seems to work magic in the whole life, gradually changing difficult mental attitudes, helping people to cope with apparently insoluble problems; giving them spiritual strength and courage to keep on.

For those who wish to work with the healing angels, the

first essential is a deep desire to be of service to humanity, and the second the ability to devote certain regular times to controlling the thoughts of the outer mind and bringing into operation the Christ light in the heart.

White Eagle says *(Spiritual Unfoldment I)*, 'Very little is known at present on the earth plane about the angels of healing, but as the age advances, many more people will not only feel their presence, they will see them. According to the need, according to the vibration created, so there come to a

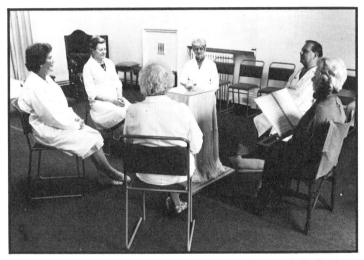

8   An absent healing group in a chapel of the White Eagle Lodge in London

healing service the angels of different colours clothed in the Light of the Sun. You know that the sunlight is full of the colours of the spectrum; now think of the angels of healing in these beautiful colours. There is nothing dark or ugly. They are all light and purity. These angel beings draw very close to the healer, who contributes the substance which they need to establish contact with those who have sought the healing power. These healing rays can be used to heal not only the physical body of individual man, but also the mind and the dark material conditions which oppress humanity.

'The radiation of the pure white magic flowed continually from the heart of Jesus. Any man can still receive in his heart this same radiation from the heart of the Christ; and if his heart keep pure and joyous it can in turn radiate light and healing to all the world.'

One essential when invoking the help of angels is stillness and calm in the emotions. Those who would heal must learn how to withdraw from the turmoil of their own thoughts and desires to the place of absolute stillness. All feeling and emotion must be so tranquil that the soul-consciousness becomes like a calm lake or sea, with the surface of the water so still that it mirrors the sky and surrounding country, making it almost impossible to tell which is the image, which the reality.

In this state of stillness we can picture either sunrise or sunset, our whole being focused on that blazing, glorious Sun-orb. It is then not difficult to imagine, coming forth from the Sun, these glorious, stately angelic beings, each one vibrant with the life and energy of one of the seven great colour rays. These are the Angels round the Throne, the Sons of the Flame, whose life-force permeates all the beings, human, animal, vegetable, mineral, which are vibrating on that particular ray. While each of these great beings is in harmony with one of the planets, their influence extends throughout the Cosmos. Their power can be healing or devastating. Learning to work with them is learning the art of magic, the magical power of thought directed by the God-will.

Sitters in the White Eagle healing groups are being trained in a safe and simple method of attuning themselves to these wonderful and powerful cosmic beings. The words of the healing service which were given by White Eagle in

183

1936 help the sitters so to calm mind and emotion that the angelic power can be invoked. As the words of the healing service are repeated constantly and regularly in the healing chapels (or the small individual sanctuaries in many parts of the world where healers are working) what a fountain of healing light and colour is built up, augmented by the tremendous power of the healing angels! When the name of a patient is called, the soul is brought, by the power of the angels, right into the heart of this living fountain. When the participants work simply and sincerely, longing with all their hearts to serve and help others, the group draws together its own band of angels, each contributing their individual colour-vibration, and every group working in this way becomes magically and mysteriously raised into the healing temple in spirit. From this temple the whole of humanity is even now held in rays of healing light, which will gradually lift the whole human consciousness to an awareness of the heavenly beings.

An understanding of the power and usefulness of the different colour-vibrations is necessary to all the healers who serve in the Lodge. The colours which we project by our thoughts, by the divine will within, are all colours of light. We can only radiate such colour through the warmth and radiance of the Christ Sun in the heart, and the finest way to project healing thought to another soul is through the heart-mind. The head-mind, the everyday mind, is limited in its ability to deal with the subtler states of consciousness. It can direct the details of the outer life; it can organise the harmony of the sanctuary; it can focus on bringing the body into a harmonious posture for meditation; but then it is best made tranquil by the harmonious repetition of the words of the healing service. The outer consciousness then quietly subsides, even as the choppy waters of a lake become still after the wind drops. Then like the rising sun over the water the heart-consciousness takes over. The colours that are used in healing radiate from this inner Sun, filling the tranquil soul with light. They are the lovely colours of spring and summer flowers, or those reflected in the facets of cut jewels. The colours of the healing angels are all clear, light, and vibrant with life-force.

Few people realise that we are constantly radiating an aura of colour according to our thoughts and emotions. The body and soul of man may almost be likened to a prism, through which the clear white flame of spirit is reflected and broken up into the different colours of the spectrum. When thoughts and emotions are calm, tranquil, kind and loving, then gentle, beautiful, clear colours will be seen in the aura, especially round the head; but as soon as negative thoughts of fear or depression come these change to dark muddy colours, gloomy and heavy. When we feel anger or temper the whole aura is filled with fiery red, a lurid, fierce and unpleasant colour; cold critical thoughts manifest as a dull steely-grey or yellow colour, not bright and glowing but heavy and dead-looking. These heavy inharmonious colours in the aura will eventually manifest in the body as a state of disease and inharmony. But when we make an effort from the heart-centre to aspire in spirit, to rise above all the turmoil and heaviness of earthly thought and feeling, it is as if a clear bright flame begins to shine in the centre of all the gloom and darkness. As soon as this light shines from the heart of the Sun within, we can call upon the help of the angels of light, the angels of healing, the Sons of the Flame. As soon as the inner spirit, growing in strength, prays for heavenly help, the angels can draw close and flood the aura of the sufferer with beautiful clear colour which disperses the murkiness and darkness. While patients can hold the contact with this light they will feel better, the disease will begin to disperse.

At present, our awareness of colour is limited to the rays of the spectrum: but White Eagle, in company with other spirit guides, assures us that in the higher realms of spirit are many more subtle colour-vibrations which are at present quite beyond our understanding. No doubt they will be discovered and used by scientists of the future in the same way as ultra-violet and infra-red rays are used at present. Colour therapy is one of the New Age techniques which will become far more widely used, especially in hospitals, in schools and hopefully in prisons; and in public buildings, especially such places as committee rooms where important decisions are made affecting many people. The science concerning the effect of colour on mind and soul is at present in its infancy, but healers will find that an understanding of the power of colour, radiated through the thought and wisely used in the environment, can be a most helpful therapy.

Our reactions to colour are peculiarly individual. There will always be some colours that we can use more easily and live with more harmoniously than others, but as we work to increase our awareness of colour and its effect on ourselves and others we will learn intuitively how to use the right colour on the right occasion. To develop awareness of colour it is a good idea to pause whenever you see one that appeals to you, one that seems to raise your thoughts above mundane matters, and then quieten the outer mind and for a few moments concentrate completely upon that colour. Breathe it in, feel that you are absorbing it into your innermost being; as though you are standing in a fountain of heavenly colour, feeling its energy, almost hearing the note of music which that colour sounds, and becoming aware of the perfume from that colour. Remain still for as long as you can and let the feeling of the colour flow through your whole being. As you do this you will begin to understand how it can be used in healing. In this way you gradually develop your awareness of the healing angels and how they use not only the colour but the radiation and the perfume of plants, and how in the mineral kingdom these angelic powers will vibrate through jewels, crystals. There is much to learn about these angelic vibrations, much knowledge which is not of the earthly mind but will unfold in the heart of those who are dedicated to the healing work and long to serve.

In a healing group where the sitters are all trying to concentrate on a certain colour to be directed to a patient, they will probably all be thinking of a different shade of the colour; but the angel of that particular ray will use the thought-vibrations of the sitters to blend the different shades in the most beautiful way; adapting the soul-power, so willingly and lovingly given, to the exact need of the patient. As a healer becomes more practised in controlling and directing his thoughts, he will be able to radiate the colours right from the heart-mind with power and concentration; and will learn to sound from his inner being the note which calls the great healing angels to augment and amplify the soul-power which he gives. For, make no mistake, spiritual healing is soul-power, and it is the Christ light within the healer which is given in service. Certainly, when the soul-effort has been made, the healing angels pour into the patient a stream of healing light and colour, far more than the healer could possibly accomplish on his own; but that soul-effort will always draw upon the healer's nervous energy, upon his life-force, and will need to be replenished. So it is wise to remember after giving healing to allow sufficient time and quiet for this life-force to flow back: which it will do, renewing the soul, if it is given time. The wise healer learns to understand his own rhythm in these matters.

White Eagle teaches that disease of mind or body is always brought about through inner conflict, through an imbalance, a lack of harmony or rhythm in the whole being. This will mean that the colours in the spectrum of the soul need bringing back into tune, and in the White Eagle healing we call upon the healing angels who work along their own colour rays to restore harmony and balance to the soul. The healing colours may also be thought of as soul-qualities which we all in time have to acquire. When the solar body is fully established, all the colours of our own individual spectrum will be so balanced that they will shine as pure white light. We shall truly be as Sun-men, radiating light, healing and strength to all whom we meet.

These colours, as soul-qualities, can be developed in meditation (see the book *Meditation*, by Grace Cooke, White Eagle Publishing Trust, 1955). To help the healer we now give a sequence of meditation which demonstrates how the patient is taken up into the healing temple, cleansed and made whole. The meditation will also increase the healer's imagination and awareness of the colours used in healing. Let us therefore become still in mind and body. Peacefully we become aware of our breathing; we listen to its rhythm until it gradually becomes slower and deeper.

The Healing Temple of the Sun

We are standing on the shores of a lake so still that the reflected light makes it look like mother-of-pearl, with soft colours gently moving, mingling with each other, ever changing. We are not alone. A shining being stands beside us, and as we breathe in the breath of God we feel as if we are enfolded in white wings of peace. Gently we are led into the lake, which is not in any way uncomfortable but wonderfully refreshing. We find ourselves swimming in the pools of different colour, being bathed in just the colour we feel our soul needs: green for cleansing; gentle blue for peace and relaxation; golden yellow for hope and vitality; amethyst to bring us consciousness of the heaven world. We enjoy the buoyancy of the water, which makes every movement peaceful and effortless, as if we are carried along by a power outside ourselves; a power infinitely loving which supports and protects us.

We look towards the eastern sky, beginning to show the rosy light of dawn; and shining brightly, a little above the horizon, is a beautiful star, the light from which makes a path across the water. All is still as we open our hearts and minds to the beauty of the morning star, herald of the day. The light grows brighter as the sun rises; and as its light grows in brilliance and intensity, our morning star seems to be united with the glory of the arisen sun. The little path of light across the water is now a golden highway. Within our heart we feel the pull of the Sun, as if we are being drawn along this golden highway above the waters of the lake shimmering below. As we come towards the Sun we begin to discern the form of a circular temple, built of a substance rather like alabaster, transparent, full of light. Tall pillars rise heavenward; and as we look up we feel very small, yet still deeply aware of the enfolding love of our angelic companion, who is now guiding us onward up seven steps to the golden arch of the entrance. Are the pillars forming the arch angelic beings? or are they stone? It is hard to tell, for as we enter this temple, this universal temple of the Sun, we are only aware of the unity of all life, of the infinite love which pervades every atom of the universe – the Cosmos. We are carried, by this feeling of love and awareness of cosmic order, right into the heart of the temple. All around us rise the shining pillars of light; and as we look up to the domed roof we see that it is formed of what appear to be angels' wings. From the centre of the dome a blazing Star shines down upon a simple white couch.

We see now that we are part of a large gathering of healers, servers both angelic and human. We are clad in white. The whole company is silently awaiting the coming of the Great Healer. The light from above grows brighter, more intense. All faces are raised towards the Star, and every soul in the temple receives a ray of light which quickens and illumines the heart, drawing forth love and worship of the Creator, the great spirit, as slowly within the Light the dear human form of the Great Healer becomes visible and solid, but radiant as if the Sun shines through Him. Especially we are aware of the beautiful hands and feet even if we cannot clearly see the features.

Each patient is brought by angelic hands to the white couch. As the healer blesses the apparently sleeping form the whole company of healers give from their hearts pure love and light. This brotherhood of healers in the Sun temple all unite as one, becoming, as it were, part of the Christ figure as he heals and blesses each individual patient. All love and power is concentrated upon the one patient, for a few minutes – for eternity. For we are outside earthly time; we are in the heart of the eternal Sun temple where all are one. At a signal from the Great Healer the angels take the sleeping patient to a small private sanctuary, of which there are an innumerable variety all round this great circular building, all open on one side to a heavenly garden. There the patient rests, enveloped in heavenly colours brought by the angel attendants. He or she waits peacefully until it is time to return to the earthly consciousness.

To this healing temple of the Sun also the angels of death bring souls whose time has come to leave the earthly life. Each soul is most lovingly brought into the presence of the Great Healer and then taken to the quiet sanctuary to sleep until they are ready to awaken to the new life which awaits them. When they wake they look out into a sunlit garden which is as dear and familiar to them as their most loved garden on earth; and thus they can walk into the sunlight to meet their beloved family and friends who are awaiting their coming.

In our hearts we are now aware of the wonderful cosmic plan which guides every life, not only in the physical world but in the infinite world of spirit where all is known, all is taken care of, by this divine Love, Wisdom and Power – the

Great White Spirit. Our hearts are therefore filled with worship and praise. As the healing session draws to a close we are aware of the song of the angels. It starts gently and softly almost as a murmur, which swells first into a melody and then harmony before it becomes an almost unbelievable chorus of praise and thanksgiving, which seems to come from every heart: every pillar, every atom of the temple joins in the glorious sound.

> 'Praise to the Holiest in the height
>   And in the depth be praise,
> In all his words most wonderful,
>   Most sure in all his ways.'

As the sound dies we know that we too must return to work on the earth plane. First let us wander for a few minutes in the infinite and eternal garden, enjoying the beauty of the flowers and trees, the song of the birds and the warm sun shining down. This is the garden of reunion where we meet and commune with those whom we love in the world of light; the garden where we come for refreshment when our physical bodies lie sleeping.

Now we must firmly return to the earthly consciousness. We breathe a little more deeply and use the will of the outer mind once more to bring us back fully into the body. We feel our feet, we move our toes, stretch our arms to bring us back to physical consciousness, becoming thoroughly aware of the earthly surroundings. Just to make sure that we are firmly back let us mentally seal the brow, the throat and the solar plexus centres with the cross of light encircled by light.

To strengthen our ability to visualise or imagine the colours used in healing, it is quite a good idea to create in the mind such a picture to which we can turn for inspiration; for instance if we return in imagination to the shore of the lake just described, just at sunrise. Feel the hush, the waiting

191

hush of all nature as the light begins to shine on the horizon. Feel this rising sun deep within your own being, feel its rays shining on the water. The sun is filling the sky and the water with glorious colour, and right in the heart of that blazing light we glimpse a human form, the shining form of the Great Healer. From the heart of the sun, under the direction of the Healer, and along the straight beams of light emerge the angels of healing. These are the angels of the soul-qualities which we all will eventually build into our solar body. See the light and colour of each angel reflected in the mirror-like surface of the water until the whole lake consists of pools of different coloured light, each under the care, under the radiance of its own angel. As you watch these heavenly sun-colours reflected in the mirror of the lake choose one, feel yourself drawn to one of the colour pools. Remember the colours are all pure and sunlit; nothing dark; nothing murky: just radiant light.

The Rose Ray

Feel yourself bathing in this rose-red pool of sun-colour; feel the cleansing, healing power of the pool permeating your soul, filling you with the divine energy, the aspiration, the strength, the joy, the courage, the creative warmth of the flame and rose and orange rays. These are the colours associated with the fire element – with angels of power and energy, and of that love which is a living creative power in the life, an inner flame of warmth and devotion. This type of love always shines in the aura as a warm rose-pink and brings to the soul a fragrance, as of one of the old-fashioned roses warmed by the sun. It is a colour which brings healing balm to souls who are lonely, bereaved, loveless, unloving, anxious about loved ones or in a state of depression and self-absorption. The warmth of the rose colour, radiating from the heart-centres of those who love, can infuse a whole gathering of people with happiness and hope, and can produce an atmosphere of happy co-operation and creativeness.

Because red is a colour of such vitality and energy, care is needed in its use, and healers are advised to concentrate chiefly on the gentle rose shades, directing these especially to the heart-centre. However, in cases of depletion, hopelessness or where there is need for courage and positive thought, the clear, more orange-red of poppies can be helpful. This should be directed mentally to the spleen, the psychic centre through which the life-force of the sun can most easily be absorbed. This colour is revitalising; it helps the bloodstream to absorb more easily the prana or life-force in the air through the breath. The rich yet gentle ruby red, directed to the feet, will strengthen these very sensitive psychic centres and also help people to find the courage to 'keep on keeping on' with their task: those who have literally or metaphorically got cold feet will be greatly helped by this. All these colours will put new heart into people who are despondent and sad.

The Orange Ray

Orange is another ray of power and warmth closely related to the reds. It is particularly helpful for a positive attitude of mind. In healing it is most often used at the spleen-centre, where it increases strength and vitality and acts rather like a tonic. Perhaps the flowers which demonstrate this colour best are marigolds, which in their warmth and vitality remind one of the rising sun. This colour is stimulating, more perhaps to the mind than the feelings, and is a specially helpful vibration for those who are engaged in mental work concerning organisation or management and who are becoming nervously tired by the responsibility. In practical life it is important to remember that these vital colours used too lavishly can be over-stimulating and tiring. They can be more helpfully used in bright clusters of colour placed at strategic points. It is good for souls who are weary or depressed to be able to feast their eyes on a small cluster of bright marigolds, a bowl of oranges, or on the pure red-gold of the evening sun reflected on still water or on distant windows. These are all colours of love and caring, but we have to remember that real love, divine love, is never dominating and overbearing; it is a gentle, enfolding radiance, uplifting, protecting, encouraging the soul to develop its own Christ-qualities in its own time.

The Yellow Ray

If you find yourself drawn to a clear yellow pool, your soul is reaching out towards divine wisdom. The angels of wisdom are so still; the yellow is really the shining yellow-white of the sun's rays. It is the colour which we see so much in spring, the clear yellow of daffodils, forsythia, celandine, all the little golden flowers of spring. This is the colour of the air element, the element which promotes communication of thought, of wisdom. Although one feels it to be a joyous, lively colour (sometimes I think spring flowers are all singing) yet as one discovers the essence of this yellow of wisdom, there is a stillness, a certainty of faith in divine love. It is the colour for those who need strengthening in faith and divine wisdom, and a good colour for those who are wrestling with mental problems, who need illumination. In the golden yellow pool, see a silver-white fountain of light, like a flame, pure, cleansing, and yet so still. Rest in this flame and the answer to your problem will be made manifest.

The Green Ray

If you find yourself drawn to the pool of green, your soul is reaching out towards the quality of sympathy, of adaptability and a practical understanding of human needs. Green is really the colour of mother earth. So much of the

194

earth is covered with green, green grass, green leaves of trees, green plants providing food for man, animal, insect, all life. What a comforting colour is green! – not tiring or over-stimulating, but gentle and cleansing. Forget now the dark heavy greens, which are of the earth, and can be depressing. Think of the lovely sunlit greens of young leaves; or the translucent, silvery green of a waterfall, reflecting sunbeams. The deepest green used in healing should not be darker than a clear emerald, which can be cooling, cleansing and soothing. Bathing in the pool of emerald will release the soul from the congestion and heaviness of material thoughts, especially when that green is bright with sunlight. This colour too has something of the quality of divine wisdom, divine wisdom organising human affairs in the most tactful, diplomatic way, bringing heavenly harmony into practical manifestation on the earth. It is the colour of perfection in matter.

The Blue Ray

If you feel drawn in your soul to the blue pool, it may be because you are in need of peace and of contact with heavenly things. The deep blue of a summer sky brings calm and peace to the restless mind; it will relax and quieten an anxious nervous system, giving a feeling of confidence in divine love and wisdom. The angels of the blue ray bring to the soul a quality of devotion, of aspiration towards divine love. Think of the blue pool with distant hills rising into a lighter blue sky. 'I will lift up mine eyes unto the hills, from whence cometh my help.' Blue indicates in the soul an out-reaching towards heavenly help which brings peace and a feeling of security even when matters on the outer plane seem hopeless. In its loveliness the blue ray is also often depicted as the colour of the robe of Divine Mother, the colour of faithful love and devotion without thought of self. The angels of the blue ray are angels of peace, that peace which comes when all fear, all anxiety for self, has faded and the soul surrenders in complete love and trust to the divine will.

The Indigo Ray

With this quality of selfless devotion which brings its own peace, we are led from blue to the beautiful and most subtle shades of indigo, violet, amethyst. These are the colours of dawning spiritual realisation, of conscious contact with the heavenly spheres. The indigo ray is again the ray of the angels of wisdom, not so much the wisdom of the earthly mind, but the unfoldment of the higher consciousness which brings the wisdom of the spheres. This is the ray of true brotherhood of the spirit which comes through an understanding, an awareness of the divine essence in every soul. It is the ray of true healing, the healing of souls by the power of the spirit. At the present time it is often through the service of healing, through training and purifying body and soul to become clear instruments for the healing light, that we come safely and surely to an understanding of the mysterious amethyst ray.

The Amethyst Ray

The amethyst ray, the ray of magic, is the ray of the true psychic. This is a ray of power associated with that most subtle of the elements – ether. If you find yourself drawn into the pool of amethyst light and become aware of the beautiful angel of this ray, you will be conscious of a blending of divine love and wisdom which is also intensely powerful. You will be reaching out towards an understanding of the inner mysteries of the white magic, that Christ magic which will eventually transform the physical atoms of the human body – the physical atoms of the whole earth to a finer vibration, which would make it invisible to our present physical sight. The *Aquarian Gospel* ('translated from the

196

akashic records by Levi'; Fowler, 1964) tells us of occasions when Jesus withdrew from the crowds just by transforming the vibrations of his body so that it became invisible, and that after the crucifixion he rebuilt the temple of his body – raised, reconstituted all its atoms, to the level of immortality. White Eagle tells us more about this in the twentieth chapter of *The Living Word of St John* (White Eagle Publishing Trust, 1979).

In the heaven-world, which is not 'above the bright blue sky', but interpenetrates our physical world, even the air seems to have an amethystine quality, rather like the slight haze on distant mountains on a perfect summer day. All magic comes under this ray, whether it is the sleight of hand of the worldly magician, or the feeding of the five thousand and the raising from the dead of a physical body. Such divine magic is the result of the mastery, by the spirit and soul of man, of all the elements of his being, bringing a perfect co-operation of the Christed man with the angels of the elements.

It is towards this end that humanity will be evolving during the coming Aquarian Age, leading eventually to that Golden Age when angels will walk and talk with men, and when 'death will be swallowed up in victory'.

The Gold, Silver and Pearl Rays

Three colours used in spiritual healing which are not in the spectrum are gold, silver and pearl. The quality of these rays is not simple but subtle. One might almost describe each one as a combination of the essence of certain healing colours.

Gold. This is different from yellow or orange yet has something of both: it is more like the metal gold, but translated into pure light. If we think first of the metal gold, gold in its purest form, shaped into a star and reflecting the radiance of the sun, we can perhaps go on to imagine, flowing through our being, a golden radiance, a healing essence which renews life, cleanses the bloodstream, washes away all weariness of soul and body. This is the most helpful colour to uplift souls who are depressed, fearful and battered by life's problems.

Silver. Just as the gold ray may be described as the essence of the spiritual life of the Sun, so the silver ray is the subtle essence of the Moon, the great Mother. Again think of the purest metal, only silver, shaped into a six-pointed star, and see it reflecting the brightest possible silver light. The actual colour could be thought of as white, only with a silver radiance. This is the colour most useful for cleansing, and for healing conditions of psychic entanglement and confusion. It can be used to create a circle of protection round the aura, or in visualising the seal of a cross of silver light encircled by that light which is used to close down each of the chakras after meditation or certain of the chakras in healing work. This colour has much to do with psychic and magical practices, and should be used with care.

Pearl. This perhaps is the most subtle colour of all and almost impossible to describe, for it contains the essence of all the colours yet keeps a character of its own. Perhaps it can best be comprehended as the Christ radiance emanating from an arisen soul, one who has passed through the full crucifixion of the lower self – the radiance of the resurrected Christ in man, a blend of sunlight, moonlight, starlight and all the heavenly colours combined, shining in a warm, human radiance of understanding love and compassion. Healers who in moments of utter dedication can be instruments for this colour will find that it sometimes has a miraculous effect. It is not an easy colour to use, for it can only flow through the heart that has forgotten self completely.

12

ASTROLOGY AND HEALING

I N CHAPTER TWO OF this book we read White Eagle's teaching about the solar body, the soul-temple, which every one of us is building while on earth. During our many incarnations we are all creating this body of light, and during each life we are learning to develop and bring into use that part of our solar body which is associated with the Sun-sign under which we were born. The work of service through healing is one way in which this happens, and it may be helpful to understand the special gifts that the Sun-signs bring to healers (and how they affect patients, too). The dates during which the Sun is in the various signs are as follows: Aries, 21 March–20 April; Taurus, 20 April–21 May; Gemini, 21 May–22 June; Cancer, 22 June–23 July; Leo, 23 July–23 August; Virgo, 23 August–23 September; Libra, 23 September–24 October; Scorpio, 24 October–22 November; Sagittarius, 22 November–22 December; Capricorn, 22 December–21 January; Aquarius, 21 January–19 February; Pisces, 19 February–20 March. The dates vary a little, however, from year to year.

If you are an astrologer you will know, when you delineate a chart, that no matter what crosses and contradictions the other planetary positions show, behind and beneath everything else shines the lesson of the Sun, which is the quality of the solar body which has to be developed and unfolded according to the Sun-sign. For instance, if you were born when the Sun was in Virgo, all the experiences of your life will be helping you to build the Virgoan aspect of your solar body. Astrological knowledge can be a great help to you as a healer, because if you know the Sun-sign of your patient, and if you can understand something of the nature of the element governing that sign (whether it be Earth, Air, Fire or Water) you should be able to understand a little of the reason for your patient's present experience. This knowledge should help you as a healer to attune yourself to the healing ray; it will give you a little key which will unlock for you a doorway to understanding of the soul of your patient. Just become quiet and meditate. Be still in mind and soul and imagine you are in the temple of healing in the inner world, with the light from the central Sun shining down into your heart. The angels of all the signs of the zodiac hold their places as pillars of light round the temple. When you feel absolutely still in this beautiful circle of the Sun, standing at the centre of the cross within the circle of light, you will find that the light will begin to shine into your mind. It comes from the heart-mind to the head-mind and you will find yourself able to interpret more wisely. Even you who are not astrologers but dedicated healers can also develop your sensitivity in this way, to help people who come to you in need.

Everyone interested in healing and serving humanity would find it helpful to become conversant with the meaning of the Sun in the signs, and with what each sign is building into the soul in a particular incarnation. The mystics of old knew how the body is linked with the signs of the zodiac, and in old books of astrology and mystical teaching you will often find pictures of the Grand Man of the Heavens, arms and legs stretched wide, and parts of the body marked with the signs of the zodiac. The heart comes under a great light shining from above, which radiates all over the body. The hands reach out to give and to serve, and the feet are firmly placed on the ground, drawing wisdom and strength from the depths of the earth.

All healers would find it useful to learn more about the

posture and poise of the physical body, not only for their own health's sake, but for their patients': because as the body is perfectly poised, as you learn to hold the head and the neck free and upright but relaxed, and to move without tension and strain, every part of the body can draw upon the energies of the heavens. Particularly interesting to astrologers is Alexander's discovery that the primary control of the body lies in the poise of the head and neck and its relation to the back, the pelvis, and the hips. It is interesting to notice how this 'primary control', as Alexander calls it, seems to be linked with the three fire signs in the zodiac. The correct adjustment of the head (Aries) leads to a straight, firm spine like a pillar of light (Leo) which leads to flexibility of the hip-joints (Sagittarius). It shows how, given good posture, the divine energy can flow freely through the physical body.

Now let us consider the great cross of the elements – of Fire, Earth, Air and Water, under which all human souls in incarnation are working and developing, and through which they work out karma on the various planes of being, for the angels of these elements are the great angels of karma, and have an important part to play in the healing ministry. White Eagle is constantly reminding us in our healing work to try to become more attuned to these angels of the elements.

1. The Fire Signs (Aries, Leo, Sagittarius)

The influence of the three fire signs in our lives slowly helps us to attune ourselves to the spiritual Sun. Healers who have the Sun in one of the fire signs can bring to their healing work a quality of faith, a quality of inner knowing. With the Sun activating the fire element, no matter what life does to you, deep down you will hold fast to your faith in God, to your knowledge of the divine Fire, the divine Light, deep within.

White Eagle has told us that the lesson which all the fire signs have to teach is that of love. But remember love is not an emotion, it is not a sentiment. Love is positive God-thought. Love is an awareness of God – God in the heart, God in the mind, God in the whole of life. Healers with the Sun in one or other of the fire signs can bring this quality of love and faith to their patients. Don't, in your enthusiasm, overwhelm your patient with hearty good cheer. Gently listen to him; encourage him to tell you his troubles, and quietly, continually, turn his mind to God, sharing with him that faith, that light, that strength and hope that you have found. Give your patients strong comforting love. Help them to build their faith, not by what you say but by your own strong assurance. It is your faith that will comfort and sustain them until their own light is stronger.

If you have the Sun in a fire sign you may find it difficult to be wise in your giving, and until you have learnt to conserve energy you may well find that you go on giving until suddenly you become completely exhausted. Learn, therefore, to withdraw in good time: to rest and relax and draw strength from nature, from the trees, from the hills, from the sea, even from your own garden. If your patient is under a fire sign you will often find that one of the reasons why he has come to you is because he too has spent his energies unwisely. Such patients feel depressed and hopeless. Give them the strength of your spirit, your own inner fire and warmth, to renew their vitality and hope. And don't be disappointed if once they feel better they rush out and dissipate their energies all over again!

Aries. The first of the fire signs is Aries, ruled by Mars, the planet of fire, and of energy, desire and will. When a soul comes into incarnation, it comes with the will to wrestle again with the problems of the physical life. The ray of the Sun (spirit) shines into the darkness, and the first sign of life is the beating of a tiny heart. The Sun rules the heart-centre, but it is exalted in Aries, sign of the head. Thus the first part of the body to develop for the new earth-experience is the brain, for the seat of consciousness is in the head. Here are placed the sense organs – eyes, ears, nose and tongue – and also the control of the central nervous system, which controls movement and touch. The fact that Aries – sign and symbol of the divine creative fire in action – rules the head should help us to realise how vital is the power of thought in creation.

If you have the Sun in Aries you will not find it difficult to think positively, particularly once you have trained yourself to still the outer mind. You have such enthusiasm for life and such a desire to *do* things, to experiment and achieve, that you may not give yourself time or opportunity to develop the true inner strength that you should be building into your solar body. If you are a healer you may have reached the stage when you long to serve, and will soon realise that your outpouring of energy needs to be tempered with discrimination. If you persevere you will be able gradually to quieten the outer mind and submit to the heart-mind. Then you will be able to visualise clearly the still flame in the heart, lightening the consciousness, and this will greatly strengthen your contribution to the absent healing work. You will particularly be able to work with the positive Sun colours – the orange, rose and flame rays. In contact healing you should be able to cut psychic links and obsessive conditions and thoroughly cleanse and seal an aura. Your sign's ruler, Mars, is the soldier of the light. The soldier of Christ carries a sword and must be very strong in the light.

Over-eagerness and enthusiasm may cause Aries patients to wear themselves out nervously so that they suffer migraines, neuralgia and painful conditions of the face; or feverish conditions requiring a period of peace and rest. The polarity with the opposite sign of Libra could give a tendency to kidney troubles. Both signs have a great need for a steadying or calming influence.

All the fire signs tend to 'think that they know', and thus must be careful not to be overbearing. Often they have much knowledge in the outer mind, but need to seek the quiet inner knowing, the inner faith which will build the confidence of the patient, not overwhelm him.

Leo. The Sun rules the heart, as we have already said; and if your Sun is placed in Leo, you may well have had some difficult lessons to learn through emotion, because you do not always love wisely. You love very warmly and whole-heartedly, with a simple, childlike trust, and you do not realise that not everyone is the same. Leo people tend to give their faith and trust too easily and then suffer disappointment. In all fire signs burns a great sense of honour and integrity. Those under the fire signs have to live in the light and cannot understand that some people have a natural feeling for secrecy, for privacy, and that there are certain matters which are better kept quiet and secret. Leo rules the fifth house, that of love affairs, children, and all creative activities. Sun-Leos love to gather round them a circle of followers and friends to entertain or organise into some happy activity. In matters concerned with children or love there may often be disappointment and heartbreak, yet this heartbreak can be a wonderful thing. If you have Sun in Leo and have suffered through your feelings, rejoice, because your suffering will open your heart to an understanding of the eternal love. This love is not sentiment but divine warmth and strength and positive goodwill which will help you to understand the deep need of your brother.

When Leo people come to you for healing, there is every reason to believe that their condition is due to heartache of some kind. You can help to awaken their understanding and their faith in divine love. As a healer your task is to open yourself to the great Sun. All healers have to do this, but with you especially it is easy to reach out to the Sun because you work from the heart and the heart is the organ of the body most readily vivified by the solar fire.

The soul working under the sign of Leo really has the task of shepherding his flock – of giving love, comfort, and strength. What a tower of strength you can be, imparting your own quality of faith in divine love, which will help your patients to solve many of their problems!

You are likely to be particularly happy using the gold ray, that warm, revitalising and restoring ray which brings strength and flexibility to mind and body. You should be able to help patients with painful backs, with arthritic conditions, and trouble both with the eyes and ears. But most of all through your own warm personality you can comfort and inspire hope and faith in them. Both in absent and contact healing, train yourself to direct the rays always from your heart, attuned to the Sun, your ruling planet.

Sagittarius is one of the dual signs, and if you have the Sun in Sagittarius you will want to learn all that you can, on the one hand, about the joys of physical life and physical activity; and on the other, you will want to reach to the stars. You want to walk, to run, to ride, to swim, to sail, to fly – oh! how you love the joy of freedom and activity!

So often when the lesson of Sagittarius is being learnt the Sagittarian experiences restriction through some sort of difficulty which affects the legs and movement generally, or through some illness which confines him for quite a long time to a chair or bed, forcing him to travel in mind and spirit rather than in body. Indeed when the body grows older and not quite so active, he will want to open his heart and mind to the mysteries of heaven; to study philosophy or metaphysics or some kind of advanced science – for the Sagittarian's mind is as active as his body is. He is often widely read and through his studies and also through intuition has attained a certain amount of wisdom. But

Sagittarians also tend to think they know, and are always ready to give advice. It might help more if they waited until the advice was sought.

The Sagittarian's restriction may not necessarily be physical. It may be in the mind, or in some tie that holds him down to work, or to family circumstances, where he can't be free. So often he has to achieve his freedom through discipline and obedience. So if you are a Sagittarian, and frustration and restriction is your lot, remember that it is there to help you to develop greater wisdom and true freedom of the spirit. Let your interest in philosophy grow, and through that, your devotion to the divine spirit. Then, because of the lovely fire element that is so strong in you, through you will come the power to heal.

Sagittarius is a mutable sign, and this means that you will have a very active and sensitive nervous system and a particularly active mind which will tend to be 'all over the place', flashing like lightning hither and thither. You must learn to hold that mind in check – this is why the discipline of the ritual of a healing group is so good and helpful to you. If you will give yourself to it, it will help you to develop your healing power and you should be able to take away pain. Because you have such faith and devotion you will be able specially to use the blue ray which is so effective in soothing pain. Blue is the colour of Jupiter (ruler of Sagittarius). When you meditate, it will be helpful for you to think of the blue sky, to be still under that blue sky. See nothing but that beautiful blue, and then create the six-pointed Star very clearly in your imagination. See it at the centre of the blue sky, and feel its light flowing through your mind and heart, and your hands if you are doing contact healing. Through that beautiful blue you will be able to soothe pain both physical and mental, but you need to train yourself to become peaceful and quiet, to restrain the fire and impatience and channel it into that beautiful blue healing ray.

2. *The Earth Signs* (Taurus, Virgo, Capricorn)

Taurus, the sign of fixed earth, is ruled by Venus, and is perhaps of all signs the most steadfast and placid. People with the Sun or several planets in Taurus seem to possess an inner strength and quietness. They stand their ground with four-square solidity. If you have a Taurean doctor you cannot but feel comforted and at peace when you are with them, for there is something rocklike in their calm, kindly composure which conveys the feeling that nothing awful could possibly happen when they are about. The Taurean gives his patients a sense of security.

This quality of reliability is found in the fixed signs of every element, but is perhaps most marked in the earthy Taurus. For this reason, if you are strongly Taurean, as a healer you should have a specially soothing and calming effect on patients who are in an overwrought, 'nervy' state. During this incarnation the ray of Venus shining through your solar body brings to your soul a deep love of beauty and harmony which you are learning to bring into physical manifestation. This is why you can bring to your patients a sense of harmony and peace, an assurance that all is well.

All the earth signs give the gift of practicality, for under their influence the soul is learning the lesson of service, learning to express in physical matter the harmony of the spheres. Taurus, the sign of the builder, gives a natural desire to build and create. Quietly and methodically Taureans will establish a beautiful home, a garden, a business organisation, a church. They like a sensible organised framework for their lives, and as they grow older they want to stay in that framework – they enjoy working in a nice comfortable rut! Some of the difficulties which Taureans meet come through their deeply emotional reaction to any person or circumstance which seems to threaten their established order of life. They become fearful, resentful, angry, and these emotions soon react on the physical health, often bringing about some kind of blockage or congestion in their system. For their healing they need the cleansing green ray of adaptability and beautiful amethyst to the heart-chakra to strengthen their spiritual aspiration and help them to adapt to change, to let go of fixed ideas and habits.

Taurus is the sign of possessions. People who have built up something want to keep it. If they build a family they want to hold it together. They accumulate possessions and tend to store things away against a rainy day, so their home, their mind, their spiritual temple can become cluttered with all the things they are wanting to hold. Many Taurean patients will come to you worried because they are forced into a situation where they must 'let go'. They are full of fear, and very gently you will have to help them by strengthening their confidence in the unchanging quality of divine love.

Taurus rules the throat. Many who have this sign emphasised in their chart bring healing to their patients through the beautiful musical quality of their voice. You Taureans may find that using your voice in singing or speaking beautiful words, such as in the Lodge healing service, releases spiritual power in you. Singing hymns of praise in a church service or chanting a mantram can help to raise the consciousness above the troubles and limitations of the physical life. As the sound, beautifully produced, vibrates through the body, it can quicken cells in the brain which enable the soul to rise above earthiness and to become responsive to the spiritual power of the cosmic healing rays.

As a healer you should be a specially good channel for the beautiful blue and green rays and the lovely turquoise of the planet Venus; also the amethyst ray of the Moon, which is exalted in this sign. Gardening would be a most helpful and restoring occupation for you, for as soon as you put your hands in the earth you will consciously or unconsciously be aware of a vital force flowing into your etheric body. The earth element is closely associated with the etheric world, and as you persevere in your spiritual service, in your healing work, you will become more aware of the etheric world and the work of the healing angels in nature.

Virgo. The second of the earth signs is Virgo, the mutable sign of wisdom, discrimination and purity, ruled by the planet Mercury. It is also a sign of psychic gifts (although if you have the Sun in Virgo you will probably say, 'Oh, I don't feel anything – I'm not psychic!'). Yet, as previously stated, the earth and the etheric world are closely related, and you too could soon become aware of the angelic life in the nature kingdom. When you are working in your garden or walking among trees, just allow yourself to relax a little and think about the devic world, about the angels of the trees and the work of the nature spirits. If you will do this (and don't think, 'it's only my imagination'!), you will slowly become attuned to them and they will help you in your healing work. You have a natural interest in herbal remedies, and in healthy diet. With Mercury so strong you are a natural student and could learn a great deal about food values, the properties of herbs, the rules of health; so as well as giving your patients spiritual healing, you will often be able to give them gentle suggestions about improving their way of life. As with all the earth signs you will want to help your patients in a practical way. Mercury rules the hands and you may well be drawn to work with your hands, through massage, physiotherapy, beauty treatment or chiropody – and of course, the traditional Virgoan profession of nursing. In all these occupations you can combine practical help with the spiritual healing. In your dedicated healing service you can become a channel for the spring green ray, which cleanses, clears congestion, and soothes inflammation. Also you can become a channel for the clear, pure yellow of divine wisdom – a quality much needed by those who are sick in mind or body.

One of the chief difficulties of the Virgo soul is uncertainty and lack of confidence. They need to overcome their fear of inadequacy. They sense a great deal; they are often closely attuned to the etheric world, yet they cannot trust their inner feelings. Being such perfectionists they are afraid of making a mistake, and so you can help your patients who have the sun in Virgo by explaining to them that there is behind and within them a greater strength, a greater light than their own, helping them to withdraw from mental turmoil, confusion and fear; and so help them to call upon this strength, this God-power in the heart. No matter what complications these souls have to meet in their outer life, their basic lesson is to learn to open themselves to the strength of the Christ. It will help them just to think of Jesus, the Great Healer, to hold the hand of Jesus and then to go forward humbly but with confidence. Just let them think of the teacher, the Master, and walk beside him in simple, child-like trust – then wisdom will flow into mind and heart, wisdom which will help them to digest their human experience and to cope with life's problems. Thus, they will begin to transmute the knowledge of books into the wisdom of the spirit. If, as a healer, you too will follow this advice, you will learn to discriminate, and to find that wisdom and purity of heart which will help you to lead your patients into harmony and perfect health.

Capricorn. The third earth sign is Capricorn, a cardinal sign, ruled by Saturn, which signifies earthly power and responsibility. In the horoscope Capricorn rules the tenth house of the career or profession. It is a sign of great determination, independence and firmness. The ray of Saturn shining through the solar body will make souls under Capricorn splendid disciplinarians both of themselves and others. Once their minds are made up they keep on steadily until the goal is reached. They know where they want to go, what they want to achieve and work to a clear and definite plan from which they refuse to be diverted. Their strength of will and determination enables them to control and direct their co-workers and they often build up a strong organisation either in the political, business, or academic world.

Capricorn and its opposite sign Cancer are both signs of power and responsibility. The Capricornian is the natural head of the family, the business group, the national or even the international group. Politicians, government officers, as well as the truly great statesmen, often come under these signs. And it seems that truly great statesmen, those who are seeking not for self, but for the good of the whole, indeed great people of any race or clime, have one thing in common. They recognise the smallness, the inadequacy, of the little personal self and are able, figuratively or literally, to go down on their knees in worship and prayer.

The beginning of spiritual service for the Capricornian, service as a healer, usually comes when wordly ambition has run its course and he no longer feels the urge to devote total energy to reaching the top materially. Then there comes instead a growing desire to devote himself to the spiritual service of humanity. By this time the habit of physical discipline is firmly rooted and it is not difficult to extend this to a spiritual discipline. As a Capricornian, once you yourself recognise the value of controlled, well-directed good thought, you will not find the discipline of your mind too difficult; and as you begin to train yourself to submit your will to the divine will, and to strive to become an instrument of light in the world, you will be able to give powerful service in healing and spiritually uplifting your patients. A wonderful strength and confidence in the divine power will flow through you and you will be able to help your patients by teaching them how to think, how to adjust their lives in harmony, how to bring into action the power of their own deeper self. One of the great gifts you can give to your patients is to demonstrate for them the power of prayer.

211

Saturn and Capricorn rule the bony framework of the body and particularly the knees. You should be able to help especially people suffering from rheumatism and stiff joints. White Eagle tells us that stiff joints really stem from tension in the mind, inflexibility and a strong self-will. You will understand this mental outlook, having experienced it; but if you can help your patients to surrender to the divine will, there will come healing through a loosening of stiffness and a cleansing of the rheumatic condition.

If you yourself suffer from stiff knees or from rheumatic complaints, you could probably be much helped by the Alexander technique, or by gentle practice of yoga postures – but under the guidance of a qualified teacher. Even more, with the power of thought, the power of the spirit, you can gradually bring light to those stiff joints. Learn how, through gentle deep-breathing, you can fill the body with healing light and draw it to any part which is uncomfortable or inharmonious. This work with thought-power, God-power, is simple but not easy. It demands steady application, but most of all it demands a constant effort gently to surrender self-will to childlike faith in divine love and goodness.

If you can convey this to your patients you will render them a great service for you will be helping them to help themselves.

As with the other earth signs you will be a good instrument for the beautiful spring green ray – you should also be able to use the silver and the flame ray, since Mars, planet of divine fire, is exalted in your Sun-sign.

3. *The Air Signs* (Gemini, Libra, Aquarius)

The air element is the subtlest of the four. It is able to permeate all the others, and astrologically is concerned with the development of the mental vehicles. By these man can be locked in the physical consciousness as in a prison, or he can rise through the higher mind to the gates of heaven.

Gemini. The symbol of Gemini, first of these signs, is rather like a doorway, a gate into a garden or the portals at the entrance to a temple. Gemini is a mutable sign, which indicates much flexibility and adaptability, the element Air at its freest and least constrained. Gemini is, of course, a dual sign, and those under its influence are likely to have experiences of duality in their lives. They often have to choose between alternatives. They may have two different jobs or a hobby which is practically as remunerative and as important to them as their official job. There is a duality in the Gemini nature too, with perhaps a rather light, superficial side, and a much deeper, thoughtful side, a side which will enable that soul through aspiration and training to touch heights of illumination. The ruler of Gemini is Mercury, the messenger of the Gods, and people with this sign strongly emphasised are usually receptive in their higher selves to impressions, ideas and inspiration from the heaven world. With training and discipline of the mind they can become attuned to angels, the angels of music, of art, of science, and they will have flashes of inspiration which they are able to translate into words, harmonies or colours which will uplift or cast down. Gemini gives the gift of easily expressing thoughts in words, of firing the imagination of the listener or reader, but the Geminian must understand how much those words affect the people around him. Healers under this sign can help and uplift their patients; or by an idle, ill-considered word, they can do just the opposite. So one of the first lessons for a healer under this sign is to watch carefully both the thoughts and the tongue.

Gemini rules the tongue and also the lungs, shoulders, arms and hands. All the air signs are closely associated with the nervous system, and some Gemini people may well suffer from tension – fibrositis; stiff, tense shoulders; or nerve troubles in the arms and hands. Also, during times of nervous strain, there could be trouble with the lungs and breathing apparatus.

Geminian healers must learn how to quieten and control their nervous system and direct the heavenly light round the body through correct breathing. This is not easy for the restless and active Gemini mind, but if the Geminian will 'keep on keeping on' with the practice of quiet deep-breathing and attunement to the heavenly places, this will quieten and steady the mind and make him receptive to the inspiration of the angels and human healers in the temple of healing.

When we consciously slow down the breathing to a gentle rhythm, and turn our thoughts to the Star of the higher self, which shines above us, we draw in the light with the air we breathe. Every inhalation fills the lungs with light, and the light penetrates the blood which is waiting in the lungs to be cleansed. This is drawn back into the heart, which is re-charged with light; and this life-force, this wonderful restoring healing power, is circulated through the whole body. But this circulation of light and life only takes place to the fullest extent when we consciously turn our thoughts to the light, and give our minds to breathing in this sustaining power.

Healers with the Sun in Gemini who will train themselves thus can become beautiful channels for the healing angels. Since Gemini rules the hands, your hands should be sensitive instruments for contact healing. You know how to touch your patient in the most gentle, soothing way. Train your mind to be still, learn not to dissipate your energy with talking and nervous excitement. Unless you keep conscious control, your tongue and your thoughts easily run away with you; and the key to this control is the breathing. Remember that Mercury, ruler of Gemini, is the messenger from God, and if you can train your mind to be still it can become a reflector of heavenly wisdom and inspiration. As you practise quiet, gentle deep-breathing, try to focus your concentration not on the brow but in the heart-centre, picturing the heart as a shining jewel with many different facets reflecting the light of the Sun. Healers with the Sun in Gemini, as they learn to rise into that higher consciousness where they reflect the light of the Sun, can powerfully direct clear radiant colours to heal the body, and uplift and restore the soul of the patient. Gemini is a sign of joy, and as you feel the joy of the heavenly contact let it flow through you to lift your patients out of the darkness of their earth-bound thoughts.

Patients with this sign emphasised may be extremely talkative, too! They are good at expressing their thoughts in words and the story of their troubles will pour out fluently. If you listen carefully you may find that after a while they are saying the same things over and over again; but beneath all the chatter you will become aware of the core of anxiety or resentment which will give you the key to their trouble. Just listen quietly and gently, remaining centred on that jewel shining in your heart, and whenever you can get a word in, try to help your patient to realise that within his own heart is a light, a strength, a healing power. In your imagination let your heart become one with your patient's heart, so that they too feel the beauty of that jewel of light. Gradually you will find that they will grow quieter and more peaceful as they become aware of the all-enfolding love and tranquillity which is flowing from your heart. Do not try to do too much. When one gets caught up in this healing work it is easy to keep on longer than the nervous strength of your physical body allows. It is true that you are only an instrument and all that you give forth in soul-power is replenished from above: but remember that this needs time and peace. If water is flowing from a tank faster than it is being replenished the tank will become empty. It is the same with spiritual and soul-healing; you need to learn how to balance

215

the inflow and outflow of the nervous strength. If you feel depleted, through unwise giving, try to withdraw quietly into natural surroundings, and breathe in the strength and healing of mother earth. You will also find relaxation in doing some form of handicraft or playing a musical instrument. It is good for Gemini people to use their hands creatively.

Libra. Now we come to Libra, the second of the air signs, a sign of cardinal quality ruled by the planet Venus. If you have the Sun in Libra your soul quickly responds to harmony or disharmony in your environment and this in turn will influence your state of health and your whole mental outlook. Your special work is to express, as far as possible, beauty, harmony and peace. Do your best to create beauty in your environment and a peaceful organisation of your activities. Libra is the sign of balance; and under its influence you are learning to hold the balance between your reason and your feelings. Thus it is hard for you to make up your mind because you always see both sides of any question – one moment you will feel the prompting of your heart, and your feelings, and the next moment reason will come up with another answer. You love thinking, balancing, comparing. Part of your work in life is to bring harmony and balance into human relationships, to smooth over difficult situations with tact and diplomacy. You are quietly intuitive and can often sense how another is thinking and, with an almost instinctive reaction, say just the right thing to put matters right.

Libra, which gives a love of beauty, harmony and peace, will also give you a gentleness of character which shrinks from argument and any kind of conflict. You would rather withdraw from a situation than fight it out, sometimes because you are so agreeable you will tend to concur in both sides of an argument and be accused of running with the hare and hunting with the hounds. Yet within you will know that in any argument no one is entirely right. To find the solution it is necessary to rise in spirit right above the problem and to wait for higher guidance; and to find this true guidance and inner strength the Sun-Libran needs to follow the same rule as the Sun-Geminian and indeed the Aquarian.

Sun-Librans who have turned from self to service and whose lives are dedicated to healing and helping humanity will be able to draw on a deep inner strength and steadiness once they have learnt how to still the activity of the outer mind. They will be able to show their patients an inner strength and steadiness and a will to overcome the inharmony in the body and soul which is causing the sickness. They will be able to help their patients hold the right thought, the creative thought of God, the thought of the Christ-power within the heart, from which all healing flows.

Souls coming under any of the air signs can be particularly helpful in any group work, as it teaches brotherhood in a practical way. Sun-Librans can help to bring that harmony and unity to a spiritual healing group which is essential to its work. It builds up the healing power in the group. Sun-Librans, dear people, are naturally gentle in their dealings with others. Perhaps their gentleness is the most beautiful quality that they can bring to the healing. When you quieten the outer mind and attune yourselves to the Star, that quality of gentleness and peace in your aura draws to you the help and inspiration of the angels of peace. You will be a good instrument for the green ray, of harmony and cleansing; and for the blue ray, which will soothe pain and calm an over-excited and disturbed nervous state. Your special gift will be to calm nervous tension and fear, and to soothe pain. Your love of beauty, expressed in your surroundings in colour or sound, will build up a healing vibration in your home which will help those who come to visit you.

The health problems of Sun-Libra patients are likely to be

217

the result of some conflict in their family or at work. Often they find themselves between two strong characters, each wanting his own way, and they are worn out, trying to keep the peace. The task of the healer is to soothe and restore the battered etheric body, and to help such patients build a circle of peace and protection round themselves. All Librans can do this with advantage. Breathe quietly, making your mind still under the Star. Then visualise a still flame. When you look at a candle you often see, round the flame, a circle of light. Now as you breathe quietly, feel yourself becoming one with that still flame, and see it gradually forming a circle of light round you. With each breath, draw the light round yourself, as you learn to do after meditation in the Lodge. Gradually you will feel that you are securely enfolded in a cocoon of light. This will protect you from the conflict and harshness of the outer life. Nothing can touch you. You are held strongly in a circle of light, yet from you can flow peace and healing to your patients.

An interesting point about the gentle sign of Libra is that it rules the kidneys and the adrenal glands, from which flows the adrenalin which gives us strength and courage to cope with difficult situations. Libra is the sign opposite to Aries the warrior, and there is always an interchange between complementary signs, so that you may well find someone with Aries strongly emphasised in the chart who has kidney trouble, or someone with Libra emphasised who will have trouble not with the kidneys but with the Arietian problems, headaches or neuralgia.

Aquarius. Now we come to the fixed air sign of Aquarius, the sign under which the human soul comes to maturity. Aquarius rules the ankles and circulation, and through its opposite sign, Leo, it can affect the heart and back. The ankles play an important part in perfect physical posture. They have to be held straight and strong so that the body is evenly balanced on the whole of the foot. If you have studied yoga with one of the Lodge teachers you will recognise the words: 'Straighten up your ankles, lift the insteps and feel the strength of the earth coming up through your body'. The perfect man stands with feet firmly planted on the earth and with the head in the heavens among the stars. As you stand erect in this way, feel the strength of mother earth rising up the body through the feet; feel the light of the heavens pouring down through the head into the heart, vitalising the bloodstream and taking life and strength to every cell of the body. Become conscious of a continual interplay between the life-force of mother earth and the light of the Sun. This is symbolised in our six-pointed Star, representing the Christed man, the human being with a perfect physical body through which Christ (the Sun) can shine.

Aquarians' great gift, even more than with the other air signs, is for group work. Often it will be they who form a group; or they will be drawn to a group formed for some altruistic, scientific or artistic purpose: but most likely altruistic, for Aquarians are naturally concerned with the welfare of others. If at a White Eagle Lodge meeting we take a census of the Sun-signs, the Aquarians usually out-number all the others, for they have been drawn by the Lodge ideals of brotherhood and service.

Because Aquarius is an air sign, Sun-Aquarians tend to live very much in the mind, in the world of thought and ideas. The strange thing about Aquarians is that although they like working in a group they are also very independent and like to get on with a job in their own individual way. They are also convinced that no one can do the job as thoroughly as they. They are probably right. Nevertheless, this independence may cause them to work themselves to a state of nervous exhaustion. Their friends may try to help, but once they have made up their minds little will stop them going their own way.

This fixity of purpose and ability to persevere is splendid

when the mind is set on an ideal, such as the radiation of the Light to help humanity towards the age of brotherhood; and this is why, if you are an Aquarian, you can be so helpful in a healing group. Once you understand what you are trying to do you can exert a steadying influence on the whole group because you can concentrate with much more strength and clarity than can the Libran or Geminian. You should train yourself to focus your whole being on the Sun–Star, to become that Light and radiate it from your heart. Then you will strengthen and uplift your patient. You may well find that work in an absent healing group is more congenial to you than contact healing, especially when you are feeling nervously depleted; but whether in absent or contact healing, you will bring to your patient a feeling of strength and steadiness. You will be able to treat a troubled disturbed mind. So many patients come to the treatment worried and disturbed about world affairs, about family matters, about their lives generally, and often they are extremely depressed. Listen as they pour out their troubles, but at the same time focus all your thought on the Sun–Star. Never try to dominate your patients mentally, but use the strength of your spirit to help them to think more positively.

Because Saturn is the traditional ruler of Aquarius you may well at times have your own battle with depression. You will think that you are being realistic and practical and can yourself become imprisoned in the negativity of the lower mind. You who are on the spiritual path know better, and you must not let yourself be pulled down by the weight of the earth. Keep a watch on your thoughts, and at the first sign of negativity, think of the light, think of the blazing Christ Star, that six-pointed Star which is so powerful on the mental plane. With all the strength of your spirit rise into that light: you can be almost like a pyramid of light. This strength that you have in your spirit is built on a four-square basis of reason. You have thought the matter out carefully and you know the truth. You must rise to the apex of the pyramid and feel that glorious Star radiating right down into the earth, into your earthly self. In that illumined state of consciousness you can be a splendid channel for the gold ray, and you may well be able to help cases of arthritis and rheumatism, and to clear conditions which come about through mental tension, over-conscientiousness and possibly through too much self-will. You will also be a good instrument for the green ray. Lift your eyes constantly to the hills: to the apex of the pyramid where shines the glorious Star which strengthens the whole of the body and mind.

4. *The Water Signs* (Cancer, Scorpio, Pisces)

Spiritually, the water element is associated with Divine Mother. It is closely connected with the emotions and with the soul-life of humanity, and all the water signs give much sensitivity, that is, receptivity to the subtler conditions in the environment. In healing work those with the Sun in a water sign must learn how to draw a ring of light and protection round their aura so that they do not absorb the psychic conditions of their patients; especially must they keep the solar plexus well controlled and sealed.

People in whose horoscope charts the water element is emphasised, or who have the planet Neptune prominently placed, are often more aware of the etheric and astral worlds than they realise, and if they are undisciplined in their use of drugs or alcohol, or over-enthusiastic in their investigations of psychic, occult or magical practices, they can easily find themselves uncomfortably entangled in elemental forces quite beyond their control.

White Eagle has often warned his students about these unwise practices, but assured them that there is no need for anyone to be fearful so long as they obey the rules of wise spiritual unfoldment. White Eagle says:

221

'There is another type of elemental outside the four ethers, earth, air, fire and water, called "astral" elementals. They are the product of man's dark thoughts when an impure condition of the physical body is brought on through a dissipated life or when the individual gives way to depressing thoughts or to severe drug-taking or drinking alcohol to excess. When these things are done it creates astral entities within and outside the aura of the individual. These can live for a long time and they are still created by the practice of black magic, as they have been created to a great extent in past ages. They eventually come back to their creator. In ancient Egypt the ritual ceremonies practised caused elementals which have lived for thousands of years. In the Druidical magic the same thing happened. They live on until they are released by love or by white light, by white magic.

'One thing we would like to impress upon you very seriously, and it is this: all elementals, whether of earth, air, fire or water, or the astral elementals created by the evil thoughts of men, are controlled by the one great Master, Christ. No man or woman need ever be troubled or hurt in any degree by any elemental entity so long as they live in the supreme light of the Christ love. There is no need to fear hauntings or unpleasant manifestations by any elemental, because you hold the mastery; that mastery is purity of motive, purity of life, and love to all creation. They will serve and will help man very much if man is living in accordance with the laws of the Master Christ.'

Cancer. The first of the water signs is Cancer, ruled by the Moon which from ancient times has symbolised the feminine aspects of life, the mother and the home. This sign is associated with the parts of the body which lie close to the heart, the breasts and the stomach. If we think of the Sun as ruling the heart, the light-centre of the body, and the Moon as the nourisher and protector of that light, we realise that

222

in every human form is symbolised Divine Mother giving nourishment to the child, the inner Christ.

If you have the Sun in Cancer it means that during this incarnation your emotional body is being vitalised and illumined by the Sun, and much of your experience will come through the feeling side of your nature. Although you are naturally practical, your real work lies in the inner sanctuary of your being, in the temple of your spirit. Here can be found the fountain of living water which will not only comfort and sustain you, but enable you to comfort and sustain others through your sympathetic and practical caring. Home and family are important to you. You also feel a deep need to build round yourself a sanctuary – even if it is only a special corner of your room, where you can retire, protected and cut off from the world. You need time and opportunity for meditation to help you to find inner stillness beneath the turmoil of worldly concerns and the clamour of the emotions. When you can touch that centre of deep peace, which is all love, healing will flow through you.

You also need to have someone or something to look after – people, animals, or plants in garden or home – and you will be happy in work which gives you the opportunity to deal with people, such as teaching, nursing, caring for the old and infirm. You like to deal with the public and could enjoy a business life, such as running a shop, or could be in a position of management in a department store. The Moon, the mother, is as much a leader in her own way as the Sun; she is the natural queen of the home, the hospital, the school, the business. Often, people with Cancer emphasised go into politics, because one's country is an extension of the home – the homeland. There is often a strong patriotism which stems from a deeply submerged memory of the peace and security of the heavenly home from which they have come into incarnation.

One of the difficulties which Cancer people have to meet

and overcome is fear: fear of the future; fear of loss; fear for the safety of loved ones; fears which can drag them down into a state of anxiety and depression and affect the health of the physical body. If you are a Cancer subject, and thus naturally receptive, you also easily absorb the fear, depression and anxiety of those around you.

In Egypt one of the loveliest paintings on Tutankhamen's sarcophagus is of Isis, with beautiful wings of protection and love outspread over the soul. In meditation you too can feel the love of Divine Mother and the protection of these great white wings, and all fear will melt away. You will know, as the Christian Scientist says, that divine love always has met and always will meet every human need.

Another symbol of Divine Mother and of the sign of Cancer is that of the tree, with roots spread wide and reaching deeply into the earth, and a strong straight trunk with branches spreading wide to shelter many living creatures. This picture would be helpful to you in meditation, for you too can learn how to draw strength from within to love and shelter those in your care. In your healing work you should find it easy to use the green ray, and also the amethyst and violet. The Moon is associated with silver, and once you are securely centred, you will be able to work quite powerfully with the silver ray, which we use to clear psychic links and entanglements. Patients under this sign who come to you for healing may well need this silver ray treatment, as they could be psychically drained by some family conflict, or by anxiety over a sick friend or relative; or they could have had some emotional shock which calls for special treatment to the solar plexus.

Scorpio. The second of the water signs is Scorpio, a fixed sign ruled by Mars. This is one of the strongest signs of the zodiac, giving deep, intense emotions with unusual powers of endurance and great courage – not quite the positive daring of Aries, the other sign ruled by Mars, for water is much more cautious than fire; but nevertheless you are a fighter, either for yourself and your own family or, later, as a warrior for the light.

Scorpio rules the excretory organs and also the genitals and the powerful sexual emotional drive. Thus Sun-Scorpios need to learn how to cope with deep and intense feelings as well as with a natural possessiveness (like their polar opposite, Taurus). They find it difficult not to be envious and possessive and must constantly be on the watch to transmute feelings of jealousy into real love and caring.

If you are a Scorpio subject, then like all those under water signs you are extremely receptive and quickly register the conditions of the people around you. You know without knowing why you know, for it is not so much in your mind as in your solar plexus that you are aware of the thoughts of those around you. You quickly feel the warmth of antagonism or friendship. As a healer you must rise above all such personal feelings and realise that you work from your innermost spirit, the light within. Learn not to be ruled by feeling and emotion and try to keep your soul unruffled as a still lake reflecting the Sun.

Unfortunately this is easier said than done, for Scorpio is ruled by Mars, the warrior, and between them they can give immense emotional energy, so that you do not entirely like things to be too peaceful and placid. There is a quality in you which enjoys coping with storms, even creating them! This is why you should find some form of work or service which is a challenge. Spiritually-awakened Scorpios need some cause into which they can pour all the strength of a selfless devotion. When that intense emotional energy is directed into selfless service it is less difficult to control temper and jealousy. Even then a constant watch must be kept, for the tongue can be sharp and wounding.

This emotional strength and devotion makes Scorpio people splendid healers. Many doctors and surgeons come under this sign. In spiritual healing you should find it easy to use the amethyst and violet rays, and also the warm rose directed to the heart. Your steadiness and determination are qualities which can help people who are depleted, who have dissipated their energy or are worn out with emotional conflicts. You should also be able to help those with nervous breakdowns if you can be patient and understanding without allowing yourself to become involved and dragged down into their emotional or psychic whirlpools. You too will be able to use the silver ray to help those caught in psychic entanglements, cleansing and clearing the aura.

You will only be able to heal in this way as you bring the emotional body under the control of your shining spirit.

White Eagle tells us, 'As the still water reflects the sky, so the calm soul reflects the image of Christ'. This is how you can help your patients. If you can become so peaceful in your feelings that your soul, like still water, mirrors the Sun, you can be a beautiful channel for the healing light which will flow through you, bringing strength, warmth, confidence and courage to your patients. Through your own inner stillness you will bring them tranquillity and peace. That inner strength of the spirit which can illumine a tranquil soul is a priceless gift to all who are sick – to your friends and indeed to the whole world.

Pisces is a mutable sign which rules the feet, the lymphatic system and the general flow of psychic force round the body. The feet are important centres of contact with the magnetism of the earth for everyone, but more especially for Sun-Pisceans. If you will stand with bare feet, spreading the toes widely so that each one makes its own individual contact with the ground, and gently take your thought down to your feet, you will become increasingly aware of the magnetism of the earth and you will begin to realise how this can give you strength and poise. Feel the weight evenly balanced over both feet, and as you breathe in consciously draw the strength and life-force of mother earth, through the feet, right up to the top of the head; then pause and become aware of the shining Star of your true self just above your head; and as you breathe out feel the purity of the light and strength from the Star flowing down through the top of your head, down the spine and legs back into the earth. If you practise the 'Tree of Light' breathing (see the pamphlet 'The Tree of Light', White Eagle Publishing Trust) in this way you will become increasingly aware of this flow of the life-forces carrying renewed health and strength to every part of you. It can be most helpful when you are feeling weary or depleted, and is a specially good practice for all who come under the water signs, for it strengthens the circle of light and protection surrounding the aura.

Pisces is another dual sign and perhaps the most psychically-receptive of them all. It is part of the special work of the Sun-Piscean to be attuned both to the heavens and to the earth plane and it is not always easy for them to distinguish between the two. Although they can be practical they also find it easy to close their eyes and ears to the muddles and difficulties of practical life and to live in an inner world of their own.

Jupiter, planet of the higher mind, is the ruler of Pisces; and like Sun-Sagittarians (also ruled by Jupiter) Pisceans have a good mind and are likely to be drawn to the study of philosophy, religion, art, music or drama. Psychic science, mysticism or occultism will all attract them. If you are a Piscean, you have a wide-ranging mind but like all subjects of the mutable signs you tend to dissipate your energies by too many diverse interests. You can also dissipate your psychic force through lack of discrimination in these matters.

You have a particularly beautiful gift for healing so long as you learn to conserve and wisely direct your energies. Many doctors and nurses come under this specially caring sign but most Sun-Pisceans prefer to work quietly in the background rather than to be organising and directing others. They like to be in a situation where their work is guided from above and where they can dedicate their life to service. A convent, monastery or a hospital is a natural home for many Pisceans because they have a deep sense of devotion and no desire to be too much involved with the conflict and turmoil of the outer world. Pisces also rules prisons, and is in polarity with the astrological sixth house (governing health and sickness); and this sign sometimes brings a physical condition, either through ill-health or particularly frustrating circumstances, which to the outer self feels like imprisonment. These conditions are of course really giving the soul a special opportunity to learn how the spirit can soar into freedom even when the body is tied to frustrating difficulties and limitations.

Jesus, the Great Healer, was the Master of the Piscean Age, and souls with the Sun in Pisces should not find it difficult to make a beautiful and powerful contact with him. The thought of Jesus, walking on the water (the emotional life) should help you, and when conditions in the physical life seem harsh and inharmonious, try to think of the Master Healer shining like the Sun, taking your hand and lifting you right out of the stormy waters so that you too are walking above them, your hand firmly placed in his. Together, you walk the path of light across the water towards the Sun. If in this way you can hold yourself peaceful and tranquil, with your soul like the calm sea reflecting the Sun, you can also reflect that sunlight of God, to heal those who are in need.

In an absent healing group you may find it difficult to focus on different colours; because of your tendency to mental vagueness they may tend to kaleidoscope, so you must try to hold your mind still and to focus clearly, but don't feel too disturbed if you cannot clearly visualise the colours. Think of the form of the Great Healer in the Sun, then try to think of yourself as being like a mother-of-pearl shell reflecting all the subtle colours of the spectrum. You should be a good channel for the pearl ray, also for a particularly beautiful soothing blue which can calm an overwrought nervous system, ease pain and bring a feeling of deep peace to the patient. You will also be well able to use the amethyst ray of divine wisdom. If you have to treat patients who are depressed and hopeless you will need to make a special effort to be positive and hopeful; and be careful afterwards to clear your aura thoroughly, so easily do you absorb the thoughts and feelings of others. When you have been treating patients or have been in contact with those who seem to draw upon your psychic strength, hold your hands under running water and clear your aura over your head and across the back of your neck by lightly flicking water over your head. Feel the drops of water coming like rays of light from your finger tips, clearing your aura, and then firmly seal the solar plexus with a silver cross-within-the-circle. Make a habit also of breathing in the light as previously described. Each morning and evening make the circle of light round your aura seven times so that you are living in a cocoon of light, through which you will be able to radiate the healing. Magically it will flow through you to heal hearts, souls, bodies and minds.

The development of the soul-qualities represented by the colours and by the zodiacal signs, through life-experience and through service, is part of the process of the creation of the solar body, described in chapter two of this book. We close with White Eagle's words from a teaching printed in the Lodge magazine (volume thirteen) under the title 'The solar force'.

'You have been told many times of the great development which is coming on the earth, when life will be harmonious and beautiful, and when men will live together in the brotherhood of the spirit. You are sometimes discouraged by what you see. When you look upon the sufferings of humanity you feel indeed you are gazing upon another crucifixion of Christ. You must not be cast down, dear brethren, but look up, and endeavour to see the vast company of shining spirits, men and angels, whose light is slowly penetrating the mists. Those unhappy conditions which distress you so much will pass. Remember they are working a purpose out in matter; and the day will come when you will be filled with joy and thanksgiving at the outworking of the divine plan.

'For you have either to accept the omnipotence and omniscience of the Great Spirit, the great Intelligence which is guiding and directing human life, or to reject and deny it.

'The basis of all religion in the future is to be brotherhood of the spirit; and later the development of a wonderful nervous system due to the quickening of the nerve-centres of the body, so that man would be responsive to the finer vibrations of life. First of all, according to the teachings of the Master Jesus, man has to find and establish in himself a consciousness of the inner light. Once this inner light is recognised and gently encouraged to grow and develop, think, my brethren, what a difference it will make! If instead of condemnation, argument and criticism, rash statements and hasty tempers – if, instead of these disturbing elements, gentleness, love and calm radiance shone through every man and woman, what a difference there would be! This indeed is what is meant by the words "At the name of Jesus, every knee shall bow". It means that every individual man striving to allow the Light of the Christ to shine through him as he goes about his business will radiate an influence which will be like the perfume of the rose; or to change the simile, it will be like an electric force in its impact upon his colleagues. The radiation from a man through whom the Christ Light shines is in a high degree identical with what is called electricity. Your etheric body is so closely related to the nervous system that it can animate and stimulate the psychic centres in the body. These centres become receptive to the eternal Sun – not the physical sun visible in the sky, but that power and light which is *behind* the sun. The nervous system of the body can become so sensitive and so attuned to the higher vibration that it can receive in great measure the electric power which has come from the inner Sun, which is indeed the source of life.

'We want you to understand that spirituality is not something quiescent, but strong and powerful, finer than the matter of earth, finer than the earth vibration. It is the substance of its life. So it is true that as a man or woman becomes sensitive to the love of God, as he desires to become Christ-like, so he brings through into physical life this power, this spiritual force. As he goes about his business other people feel this force, rather as you see a light which is switched on in a room. The person who has the inner Light takes that Light wherever he goes. Thus it is that the vibration or *name* of Christ – the vibration *is* the name which sounds throughout the earth – is the vibration of Light, or of this highly refined electricity, and is felt and seen. People do not understand its nature, but they recognise that certain people seem to bring healing or a light as they enter a room. Those who recognise the light instantly acknowledge it. They bow in their souls, in their minds; they recognise something, they acknowledge it. In this way they bend the knee to the vibration of Christ, the Son.

'You look forward to the Second Coming of Christ, for it is said so clearly that he will come again. You have heard us say on many occasions this Second Coming will be in the heart of every man and woman. It will be the awakening of the light. When this light burns bright in the human soul, then will come about the refinement of the nervous system. First of all the purification of matter, of the physical body, the earth. Then will come the control of the next body,

231

which is the emotional, the desire-body. After that, perhaps, a greater task still, will come the control of the mental body – the mind-body. After that will come the birth of the divine, the Christ-man. The Moon represents the mind-body, the Sun represents the spiritual body. Before man can attain mastery over this earth there must come about the marriage or perfect union between the mental and the spiritual body.

'There is a great deal to learn, my brethren. A world of unfolding beauty will open when you take the trouble to tread the path, proceeding by the way of meditation, prayer, devotion; not by ostracising yourself from man's life, but by living in the world as a son, a daughter of God. Meditation will take you right up through all the planes into the heavenly Light, into that celestial world of the perfected sons and daughters of God. *Eye hath not seen, nor ear heard the things which God hath prepared for them that love him.* This, my brothers, is the path which the Aquarian Age opens up, beauty and harmony and brotherhood from earth to heaven. Then Jacob's ladder will be raised upon the earth and every seeker whose vision is quickened will see the angels coming and going 'twixt earth and heaven. You will learn for yourself that we speak the truth. We cannot give you proof, but the proof is waiting for you to find in your own evolution. Do not be content to listen to our words or to read the writings of the initiates and mystics and sages. *Seek truth for yourselves*, and you will surely find the jewel, a treasure of great price.

'God bless you. May you receive God's blessing – now.'

NOTE

Readers and healers who feel they would be helped by a greater knowledge of astrology may wish to have their horoscope cast by the astrologers of the Lodge, or may wish to study the subject themselves through the White Eagle School of Astrology.

The natal horoscope delineated by White Eagle astrologers gives soul advice and guidance of an intuitive nature as well as a full character analysis. It is suggested that you write in the first instance for an application form and details of costs, to the White Eagle School of Astrology, New Lands, Rake, Liss, Hampshire GU33 7HY. A briefer but nonetheless very carefully prepared computer analysis is available at less cost from Rose Elliot Horoscopes: for details write to the White Eagle Publishing Trust.

Instruction in the White Eagle School of Astrology is by correspondence course, prepared by Joan Hodgson, and there are also regular meetings and lectures in London and in Liss, Hampshire. The three courses are designed to guide the student from the earliest stages to become a profession-ally qualified astrologer, and culminate in a Diploma examination.

The beginners' course starts from first principles and is so simple and clear that anyone with interest and determina-tion can successfully calculate a chart and give a simple interpretation by the time they finish the twelfth and final lesson. The intermediate course is for students who already know how to calculate a chart. These six lessons take such students to the point where they are ready for the advanced course in horoscope delineation. The advanced course makes a thorough study of the interpretative side of astrology, including rectification, vocational guidance, chart comparison, health, karma, and the deeper spiritual aspects of the chart. For details of these courses you should write to the address above.

REFERENCE GUIDE

THE STARS AND THE CHAKRAS

Joan Hodgson

Joan Hodgson's most recent book. While its predecessors have concentrated on self-understanding through astrology and meditation, THE STARS AND THE CHAKRAS takes their theme into a new dimension. It shows how the divine spirit took on human form that it might grow—roll back the darkness, as it were. Through life-experience, the soul finds its way back to Oneness, to God.

Joan shows that through astrology this process can be clearly described. The sequence of the planets (in particular) illustrates the descent of the soul into matter and its eventual arising into the sunlight of God, for the same sequence recurs in the planetary rulership of the chakras, or spiritual centres, in the human body.

Much has been written about opening the chakras and in particular of raising the basal fire, the *kundalini*. Joan shows that this is a completely natural process which life itself teaches. The greater awareness that comes through the study of spiritual teachings simply brings the acceptance necessary to make this process easy.

As humanity moves forward into the Aquarian Age, the individual becomes motivated by thoughts of brotherhood, of drawing together with other souls in groups for service. This too is demonstrated in the stars, as a result of one of the most important astrological discoveries of recent years: the thirteenth zodiacal sign of Arachne. Arachne, the spider, draws out the deeper meaning of life for each soul and spins her web, pulling individual into brotherhood with individual, working for the development of the group consciousness.

Joan is able to take a special example of this from her personal experience: the founding, under instruction from spirit, of the White Eagle Lodge. It is a fascinating and evidential story. And so in THE STARS AND THE CHAKRAS she leads the reader forward and backward through time in a great meditation on human life: back to the ancient ceremonies of the sun temples and forward into the universal consciousness, towards which the new age draws us.

181 + xi pp, hardback, diagrams, 216 x 138 mm
ISBN 0-85487-082-2

WHITE EAGLE'S
'SPIRITUAL UNFOLDMENT' SERIES

Four books of White Eagle's teaching which show how by the growth of the soul-understanding man can truly contact higher realms of spirit and serve creation, thus entering into the full richness of life.

SPIRITUAL UNFOLDMENT 1

Subtitled 'How to discover the invisible worlds and find the source of healing', the first volume sets out a simple way of spiritual unfoldment that is practical and rooted in everyday experience.

137 + vii pp, hardback, 186 x 123 mm
ISBN 0-85487-012-1

SPIRITUAL UNFOLDMENT 2

'The ministry of angels and the invisible worlds of nature': this volume shows how man can learn to see into and co-operate with the angelic and devic kingdoms.

103 + ix pp, hardback, 186 x 123 mm
ISBN 0-85487-001-6

SPIRITUAL UNFOLDMENT 3

'The way to the inner mysteries': a re-awakening of memories of the mystery schools of old for all students on the spiritual path.

114 + xiv pp, hardback, 186 x 123 mm
ISBN 0-85487-075-X

SPIRITUAL UNFOLDMENT 4

'The path to the light': completing the series, this book looks forward on the spiritual path as the soul gains wisdom and begins to balance its opposing aspects. 'You walk the path from the unconsciousness or darkness of the human life into the glory and light of the divine.'

116 + xii pp, hardback, 186 x 123 mm
ISBN 0-85487-078-4

THE LIVING WORD OF ST JOHN

White Eagle's Interpretation of the Gospel

The gospel of St John is separated from the other gospels by the profoundly mystical quality of its teaching. This applies particularly to the account the Master Jesus gives of his mission on earth and of his own relationship to God.

White Eagle's interpretation is in this mystical tradition, and is a meditation on the truth which the words of St John the beloved so beautifully convey. The most important message of this book is that the Christ is the central life, or light, within each one of us, and that the path which Jesus trod is the same slow road that each of us takes, over many incarnations, until we too become as 'man made perfect'. The keynote of all religion, White Eagle would say, is love.

Readers used to the esoteric tradition will find in these pages an exposition of the gospel which implicitly harmonises the religions of East and West, and makes the old boundaries seem altogether less relevant. More orthodox readers of the gospel will find that the spirit of it is refreshingly alive as White Eagle expounds it.

White Eagle's interpretation was largely given in talks to a group of his students in the war-torn London of the forties, but the present edition contains much teaching given since then which broadens and completes the vision.

194 + xiv pp, hardback, 234 x 156 mm
ISBN 0-85487-044-X

THE STILL VOICE

A White Eagle Book of Meditation

A selection of readings from White Eagle's teachings, leading into meditations for individual daily use, or for use by groups. It brings a new understanding of brotherhood, service, and the oneness of all life. A perfect companion whenever peace of mind is sought.

ISBN 0-85487-049-0
113 + xv pp, hardback, 165 x 102 mm

WISDOM IN THE STARS
Joan Hodgson

This classic book on astrology is one of the simplest introductions to the subject that could be found, for it is simply an account of the destiny that accompanies each of the Sun-signs, from Aries to Pisces.

In their deeply meditative form, however, the twelve chapters will be of help to even an advanced astrologer; while anyone seeking to understand life from a spiritual perspective, even if not an astrologer at all, will find their vision and awareness opened by it.

'Joan Hodgson's beautifully simple, smoothly flowing style reveals a depth of understanding fully commensurate with her long experience as an astrologer' *Astrological Journal*

116 + xii pp, sewn paperback, 178 x 111 mm
ISBN 0-85487-030-X

WHY ON EARTH
An Introduction to the Ancient Wisdom through
White Eagle's Teaching

Joan Hodgson

The commonest cause of suffering is the ignorance that *man is spirit* in a mortal body, and that spirit is free, deathless, and as divine and living as its origin. This is the central principle of White Eagle's teaching and of the Ancient Wisdom, knowledge expressed so simply in the teachings of the Master Jesus.

Joan Hodgson first wrote this book to provide young people with an introduction to White Eagle's teaching, but it has proved of value to people of all ages seeking deeper answers to the stresses and sometimes tragedies of life.

'Problems are handled compassionately' *Alive*

133 + xi pp., sewn paperback, 178 x 110 mm
ISBN 0-85487-043-1

PLANETARY HARMONIES

An Astrological Book of Meditation

Joan Hodgson

This book gives a new dimension to the practice of meditation by identifying the planetary influences which are at work at any time of the day, or at any time of the lunar cycle (the month) or the solar cycle (the year). Joan shows how the planetary movements affect our lives and how meditations which are linked to them can bring a unique peace and blessing. The cycle of meditations that she gives resembles the well-known Essene communions in its recognition of the angelic presences at these times.

As an astrologer Joan is also able to give guidance to the individual about meditation, because the Sun-sign of the individual brings its own qualities to the meditational practice.

Constant communion with the Sun and the heavens is the perfect way to attunement to the great rhythm of life and to our own planet.

The two-colour illustrations by Margaret Clarke complement the text by bringing the natural world closer as one reads.

145 + xv pp, illustrated in two colours, hardback
ISBN 0-85487-081-4

HEAL THYSELF

White Eagle

A way for everyone, sick or well, to find and retain true health of mind and body. The higher self knows no limitation, and through it flows the Christ healing and radiance which can melt away all ills and resolve all difficulties.

55 + ix pp, hardback
ISBN 0-85487-015-6

ASTROLOGY, THE SACRED SCIENCE

Joan Hodgson

A book about the destiny of man, in astrological terms, for all who ask the basic question about life on earth. It describes the Cosmic Cycle by which souls come into incarnation after incarnation, the zodiacal and planetary influences which shape their characters, lives and bodies, and it gives a visionary account of the Aquarian Age and of the Ages in which man slowly rediscovers the consciousness of God.

ASTROLOGY, THE SACRED SCIENCE, now one of four books Joan has written on esoteric astrology, deals principally with the Seven Rays of unfoldment and with the planets associated with them. More than this, Joan treats the human being as a microcosm of the 'Grand Man of the Heavens', endowed with all the elements of perfection within himself, only waiting for growing consciousness to bring them into manifestation. She thus describes not only the individual's path to perfect awareness, but the Great Cycle of human destiny.

'An inspiring volume on esoteric astrology, bringing forth insights and revelations we've not read elsewhere' *The Yes! Bookshop Guide*

'It is not often that I feel at a loss for words, but this book seems to me ... in a class by itself, not just because it is beautifully written and is so much more than just another book about astrology. It succeeds in demonstrating the spiritual law of the cosmos. I know of no writer better qualified to expand on the Seven Rays. A must for any student, however uninformed technically about astrology, for its introduction to spiritual truth' Ingrid Lind in *Prediction*

238 + xviii pp, sewn paperback, 216 x 138 mm
ISBN 0-85487-046-6

YOGA OF THE HEART

A White Eagle Book of Yoga

This is a very practical guide to the postures of yoga—but one which, by giving their inner meaning and effects, adds a whole new dimension to them. YOGA OF THE HEART uses the words of a Western spiritual teacher, White Eagle, to bring into harmony the deep and very beautiful philosophy of yoga and the European traditions. At heart the Christian message and that of the classical yoga teachers is the same: love for all beings, including kindness to oneself.

This is therefore a book which enables us to practise yoga at the deepest level, at which more than just physical health is achieved. Through yoga, inner tensions and psychological worries are brought naturally to the point of release. Jenny advocates the use of affirmations as an additional help in this. She shows how the choice made in the heart and the mind affect the physical body and, through the postures, can be used to bring change in the life. Throughout all this, the practice of yoga allows a focus upon God to develop—and this, in time, brings the deepest happiness.

Special features of this book are the chapters on yoga in pregnancy and for those to whom physical handicap or illness gives a special opportunity to benefit from yoga practice. Jenny includes suggestions for a personal practice programme for everyone. The selection of postures also covers all those needed for the Iyengar Introductory Teachers' Certificate.

The *asanas* are illustrated at each stage, and the book is designed to stay open for ease of reference during practice. As a source of further assistance, four tapes by Jenny Beeken, covering most of the postures in the book, are also available from The White Eagle Publishing Trust.

large landscape-format hardback, 189 x 246 mm
ISBN 0-85487-080-6
178 + xiv pp, 177 illustrations,

THE QUIET MIND
Sayings of White Eagle

All the sayings in this treasured little book catch White Eagle's unforgettable tone of voice.

THE QUIET MIND has provided many people with their introduction to the White Eagle teaching.

(POCKET EDITION)
90 + vi pp, hardback, 117 x 89 mm
ISBN 0-85487-009-1

(LARGE-PRINT EDITION)
90 + vi pp, hardback, 202 x 130 mm
ISBN 0-85487-060-1

BEAUTIFUL ROAD HOME
Living in the Knowledge that You are Spirit

White Eagle

In this, the most recent White Eagle book, the loved 'gentle brother' seeks to remind his readers that they set out many incarnations ago upon an absolutely safe journey: the path of the unfoldment of their spirit through the experience of everyday life. Far from life being punishment, the reality of the whole of life is light, love; and it is only our dimmed awareness that perceives the world and ourselves as heavy, physical.

Development of the awareness brings happiness, for then we see not with the limited eyes of earth but with the fuller understanding of the heart. Life becomes not an endless struggle but ... a beautiful road home. This is a book of the deepest comfort and inspiration.

84 + xii pp, sewn paperback, line illustrations, 202 x 130 mm
ISBN 0-85487-088-1

MINESTA'S VISION

A Centenary Collection of Grace Cooke's Writings

The life of Grace Cooke (1892-1979)—'Minesta', as she is known in this book—was one that touched many other people's. Her gift of clear vision gave her a perspective on human existence that enabled her to see what others believed they could not. From the age of twelve she was able to use this gift in a way that could totally transform the attitudes of others towards the conditions of their lives. Yet this gift was coupled, not with any sense of being someone special, but simply with a warm awareness of the role of mother. Through her gentle mediumship came words of great wisdom—White Eagle's; the relationship between them is one of the underlying fascinations of this book.

It contains extracts from her writing over many years. There is one complete and otherwise unpublished teaching by White Eagle in which he talks of himself and his instrument, and there is a clear glimpse of her human qualities active within the organisation that she founded under his guidance, the White Eagle Lodge. First and foremost, however, it is a celebration of *her* writing, less often heard, at the time of the centenary of her birth.

We can share with her in this book a truly sensitive attitude to nature, heightened by her clear vision, which enables her to reveal to us this invisible world; we can re-live with her the beauties of the Western Isles, notably the Iona she specially loved; we can understand, from her writing, the inspiration White Eagle's teaching offered to those who sought to understand the experience of the second world war; we can share with her, most closely, the realisation of her vision in the building of the White Eagle Temple at Liss in Hampshire: truly 'a meeting place between this world and the next'. Her own life is described with great humanity in the editorial text, and although this is not intended as a biography, a very real picture emerges of her qualities, her struggles, and above all her service to her human brothers and sisters.

56 + xiv pp, wire-stapled, line illustrations by Cloda Whyte, large format, 202 x 202 mm
ISBN 0-85487-089-X

All the books mentioned are available from:

THE WHITE EAGLE PUBLISHING TRUST

NEW LANDS · LISS · HAMPSHIRE · ENGLAND

THE WHITE EAGLE PUBLISHING TRUST is part of the wider work of the White Eagle Lodge, a meeting place or fraternity in which people may find a place for growth and understanding, and a place in which the teachings of White Eagle find practical expression. Here men and women may come to learn the reason for their life on earth and how to serve and live in harmony with the whole brotherhood of life, visible and invisible, in health and happiness.

Readers wishing to know more of the work of the White Eagle Lodge may write to the General Secretary, The White Eagle Lodge, New Lands, Brewells Lane, Liss, Hampshire, England GU33 7HY (tel. 0730 893300) or can call at The White Eagle Lodge, 9 St Mary Abbots Place, Kensington, London W8 6LS (tel. 071-603 7914).

In the Americas please write to the Church of the White Eagle Lodge, P. O. Box 930, Montgomery, Texas 77356, and in Australasia to The White Eagle Lodge (Australasia), Willomee, P. O. Box 225, Maleny, Queensland 4552.